ADVANCE PRAISE
FOR *JOURNEY TO CENTER*

"More than anyone I know, Tom lives what he teaches, and once again with rare wit and insight, Tom teaches us lessons of life that continually add value and that magically bring me back home again, to center. *Journey to Center* is a must-read."

—*John Denver*

"Centering is the art of being fully alive, and I would recommend no one to be your guide in this important journey more than Tom Crum. *Journey to Center* is a book that will be very important in your life."

—*Ken Blanchard,*
coauthor, The One Minute Manager

"Tom Crum put his heart and soul into this book. It is an easy read, but very rich in content. I am proud to call Tom Crum a friend and I highly recommend *Journey to Center* to anyone who needs to move toward *Center* and lead a richer life."

—*Charlie Eitel,*
President and Chief Operating Officer, Interface Inc.

"Tom's artistry as a storyteller and his humble, generous spirit come together to lead the reader on a fascinating journey to center. This lively and compelling personal account offers interpretations of a profound topic—that of moving through life from a center-point which radiates calm, confident inner strength. Anyone who is interested in developing a powerful center should read this book."

—*Ginger and Hiroshi Ikeda*

ALSO BY THOMAS F. CRUM

The Magic of Conflict

A Fireside Book

Published by Simon & Schuster

Thomas F. Crum

Journey to Center

Lessons in Unifying Body, Mind, and Spirit

FIRESIDE
Rockefeller Center
1230 Avenue of the Americas
New York, NY 10020

Designed by Katy Riegel
Manufactured in the United States of America

3 5 7 9 10 8 6 4 2

Library of Congress Cataloging-in-Publication Data
Crum, Thomas F.
Journey to center: lessons in unifying body, mind, and spirit/Thomas F. Crum.
p.   cm.
1. Self-actualization (Psychology) 2. Centering (Psychology) 3. Body-mind centering
4. Crum, Thomas F. I. Title
BF637.S4C77   1997   97-25840
158.1—dc21   CIP
ISBN 0-684-83922-9

To Tommy, Eri, and Ali,
on their own journey to center.

Acknowledgments

A deep bow of thanks to a cast of wonderful guides: to my own brilliant in-house editor and lifelong partner, Cathy Crum, without whom this book would be 3,000 pages long and useful only in the smallest room of my house; to Judy Warner, Aiki Works trainer and director of our New York office, whose organizational, cattle-prodding, and deciphering skills somehow kept this manuscript together despite the fact that I often wrote it on tiny yellow Post-it pads and truck-stop napkins; to Major Hal Bidlack, Ph.D., U.S.A.F., who used his years of disciplined, regimented military intelligence to keep this book funny, witty, and irreverent; to my Simon & Schuster editor, Sarah Pinckney, who, despite all of her talents, has still not broken free of N.Y.C. to go skiing with me in Colorado; to a group of wonderful friends and colleagues for their invaluable tips and suggestions: Gail Hammack, Jeanie Tomlinson, Judy Ringer, Glen Dutton, Pam Stacey, Karen Valencic, Rio de la Vista, Jeff Finesilver, Ellen Stapenhorst, Jane Lawson, Rod O'Connor, Puja Dhyan, John

Phillips, Weems Westfeldt, and Maggie Jones. And a special thanks to Ram Dass, whose wonderful teachings through story-telling over the years have been an inspiration to my work. And finally to all my family, friends, and students, without whom the experiences in this book never would have happened.

Contents

Contents

Introduction

I am a teacher. I once thought I taught many things. I taught mathematics. I taught martial arts. I taught skiing. I taught conflict resolution and stress management. Not too long ago I realized that I didn't really teach *many* things. Only one. I study and teach the art of centering. Joseph Campbell once suggested that we are not searching for the meaning of life. We are searching for the experience of being *alive*. Centering is the art of being fully alive. And wherever the art of centering is practiced, things change dramatically.

Once after a three-month-long meditation training in the Swiss Alps, I was skiing near my home in Colorado. I paused to center on a sunny rock. When my eyes opened again, everything looked so different. Was it because I had been overseas for so long, or was it something else? The diamond sparkles reflecting from sun and snow, the delicate beauty of the orange and red flora decorating the rock's surface, my ski poles standing in the snow, framed a mystical scene of clouds and mountains, the arms of heaven and earth intertwined. I was like an infant hypnotized by a dangling mobile.

Sitting on my rocky perch looking out over those familiar slopes, I noticed an old man slowly weaving his way toward me. I could see that this was not an ordinary skier. The sparkle in his eyes and the curl of contentment on his lips showed a person fully present—connected, alive, aware. He may have been more powerful in his younger days, but I am certain his artistry and his presence were never more evident. He planted each ski pole delicately and purposefully, and flowed into each turn as if saying "Yes!" to the mountain. He was beyond caring what others thought. He was simply there, present and joyful. He was centered.

Centering is not an abstract term, but rather a practical tool available to all of us. We each have the ability to unify body, mind, and spirit in a manner that will make us more relaxed, energized, and integrated than ever before. We can release stress rather than acquire it. When we center, it manifests in harmonious relationships, peak performance, heightened awareness, and creativity. The old skier was a study in energized awareness. He was *of* the mountain, not just on it. This book will shed light on what that means and how to do it.

Centering happens as the mind, body and spirit begin to align. Our muscles noticeably relax, our body straightens, clarity of thought and action become more prevalent, and vitality builds. Centering is not a stoic tightrope through life keeping us from our feelings and passions. Instead, centering is a spacious field in which we can embrace emotions and events with awareness and compassion. Centering will allow us to fully feel emotions and will at the same time give us the strength to take action not from the ever-changing weather patterns of emotions but from our highest purpose.

14

We have each had the experience of being centered hundreds

of times in our lives (often without being mindful of it). Centering happens in shades, in degrees of intensity. We don't have to be perfect about it, because each shade makes a difference. Centering is "the zone" spoken of by great athletes. It can also be a barefoot run on the grass on a summer's eve, with the wind in your face and the senses wide open. Center is a focus so present that time seems to stop as it does for a child at play. Center is a connection so deep that there is no separation between subject and object, an awareness so heightened that beauty and truth, the form and formless, melt together. It is like a delicate flower growing out of solid rock. Center can be a cosmic laugh rippling out to the ends of the universe. It can be simply relaxing in rush-hour traffic. Center is returning home. It is always a choice we can make.

This book is a storybook, a series of adventures about my own journey to center. People may forget theory, concepts, and suggestions, but rarely do they forget a good story. At the end of each chapter I offer ideas and suggestions to help you on your own journey to center.

In my first book, *The Magic of Conflict,* and in the various programs on conflict management, optimum performance, and skiing that I lead for organizations and the general public, I devote much time to the teaching of centering. I often draw from by background as a student and teacher of the graceful martial art of aikido. In my workshops, I teach the participants a variety of physical and mental exercises, some of which I have included in this book, to support them in beginning their own practice of centering. Through centering, we can turn a life of work into a work of art.

Centering works!

I have taught centering skills to audiences as diverse as elementary school students and the top management of major corporations. It's quite a sight to see one thousand uniformed Air

Force Academy cadets or a hotel ballroom full of seasoned Wyoming cattlemen standing together and enjoying the practice of center.

Anyone can return to center no matter what the situation. When I teach the employees of a major corporation how to practice centering techniques, they are creating an environment in which enthusiasm, awareness, and quality follow naturally. They automatically begin to align as a team. Centering is enjoyable and valuable at the same time.

The first section of the book, "Aha!" is about those magical moments when the importance of center became glaringly obvious. It is as much about falling off center as it is about being centered. In either direction great learning takes place.

Do you want to be centered all the time? I know how to do it. Stay in a comfy bed. Or, better yet, stay under your bed and only have those persons who love you unconditionally serve you. You may be centered, but you'll live a terribly unfulfilled life. A far more satisfying life would be to add value to the world and to learn and grow from it. Falling flat on our faces is an integral part of that process. Life is painful at times, but there is a distinction between suffering and pain. Suffering results when, after we've been thrown off center, we wallow in the mud of our self-judgment and forget to get up. As you will see in the stories that follow, I'm in the mud a lot.

The second section, "Uh-oh!" concerns the difficulties of centering in our daily lives: in relationships, at work, and at play. The choice to return to center is where some of our most intense learning takes place. In returning to center we become aware of the stumbling blocks that tripped us up in the first place. Things like ego, cluttered thinking, greed, laziness, or anger. Little things.

All right, so those aren't such little things. But they sure do show up in life's little happenings—a judgmental look from our employer, a red light in rush-hour traffic, the sudden ringing of a telephone, or the dog leaving a gift on the carpet. No big deal, right? But those little things can throw us way off center. And there's our opportunity!

For example, we can learn to take a moment during the first ring of the telephone and at every red light, to settle down, breathe deeply from the abdomen, and get centered. All of life's little upsets are simply bells to remind us to get centered and to smile at life.

Our centering ability grows with practice. And isn't life itself the ideal practice time? The challenges and chaos that we live in can be the sandpaper to smooth out our rough edges. And centering is a tool to help us get the job done with maximum joy and minimum effort. Life is worthy of our awe, our focus, and our laughter. A Christian monk, Brother Lawrence, once said, "It is not necessary to have great things to do. I turn my little omelet in the pan for the love of God."

The third section, "Ah, Yes!" deals with the significant transitions of healing, relationship, dying, and death. We are immersed in a world of major transition, both planetary and personal. Many of us are confused about our profession, our relationships, our purpose, our world. By staying busy, we can avoid taking a deep look and unveiling the truth about our cluttered lives and deepest fears. We can hide from the confusion, the uncertainty. But we do have a choice. We can be courageous enough each day to go *inside,* to our own center. We can discover who we really are and take a stand on our deepest values. This is how we mindfully live a life of center.

Center is about accepting the pressures of life. Center is about inviting change, not mindlessly holding on to a position. It takes courage to change our perspectives. It takes courage to examine which beliefs really work for us. It takes guts to get off a limiting, but often comfortable, point of view and shift to a larger viewing point. When we're lost in a densely wooded area, it helps our perspective to move to higher ground. This enables us to witness our position—not in isolation but in relation to everything around us.

We can all learn, each moment, to pierce through our cluttered thoughts to a higher purpose, and journey to higher ground. It is a path of learning and magic. It is the center of the storm.

Part I

Aha!

Nothing whatever is hidden;

From of old, all is clear as daylight.

The old pine-tree speaks divine wisdom;

The sacred bird manifests eternal truth.

There is no place to seek the mind;

It is like the footprints of the birds in the sky.

Above, not a piece of tile to cover the head;

Beneath, not an inch of earth to put one's foot on.

Sitting quietly, doing nothing,

Spring comes, and the grass grows by itself.

If you don't believe, just look at September, look at October!

The yellow leaves falling, falling, to fill both mountain and river.

—Zenrin

Center of the Storm

*The path through the wilderness begins
with the breath—deep and full.
Inhale calmness, exhale awareness.*

I was alive. More important, I was *still* alive. I was breathing. That was enough. It had taken a crisis, but I was awake. Looking out the hut window at big fluffy flakes falling lightly on the pine trees brought joy to my senses. The crackling fireplace in the background warmed my spirit.

The day had started out ideally. John and I had skied cross-country about nine miles through the dramatically stunning Colorado Rockies to a wilderness hut tucked neatly into a mountainside over two miles above sea level and eight miles from the nearest town. The day had been crystal clear, following an evening storm that had painted the earth brilliantly white with eighteen inches of fresh powder. When we arrived at the hut, our depleted energy level magically returned. We noticed the seductive slope above the hut. It was beckoning to be skied.

Sure we were tired. It had been uphill all the way thus far. Why not one more push to the top of the "knob" for an ecstatic powder run down to a cozy hut and hot dinner? Sure, the day had grown ominously darker. But we could see the top, our "skins" were already on our skis ("skins" are a long piece of synthetic material that automatically glues to the bottoms of your skis, giving you the traction necessary to ski uphill), and the lure of powder had us hooked. We quickly threw our heavily laden backpacks into the hut to lighten our load for the day's last run.

Skiers often talk about "that last run" as the one you have to watch, as the one to avoid. It had always sounded like a funny theory to me. Is it ever possible to avoid your last run? I mean there is always a "last run," whether it's at noon or at 5 P.M. In truth, the only way to avoid your last run is to not take any runs, which may save you from an injury but provides you with a rather empty ski trip. But my rejection of the "last run" philosophy did not exactly add credibility to my judgment about being out at dusk with a winter storm settling in, clad in a light windbreaker and a cocky attitude. Maybe it's the addiction to untracked powder that numbs reason and dulls years of wilderness experience. The lure of the silence as your skis rhythmically porpoise in gravity-free flight through clouds of powder can color the sanest judgment.

Being within shouting distance of your buddy is critical in wilderness skiing. There is no ski patrol to call, no groomed trails, no marked terrain, and darn few fast-food outlets. In the wilderness, beginner slopes can become the most difficult double black diamonds after only a couple of turns, with creek beds, avalanche chutes, logs, and trees lurking in the sea of white. So the buddy system is a must. A holler or yodel is the blessed sound of security in wilderness skiing. Unless, that is, you don't get one back.

John was my buddy, a trusted partner in wilderness ski trips. As we slowly climbed to the top of the mountain for our last run, the snow began falling heavily. When we reached the top, visibility was poor. We removed the synthetic skins from the bottoms of our skis, freeing the boards to do what they do best—go downhill. My fingers were numb and my face felt the bite of the wind. I looked forward to the fireplace and the hot chocolate waiting in the hut below.

Because of poor visibility we decided to change our path from the open route that led directly to the hut, to a route through the trees to our right. Our choice was steeper and densely forested, but we knew the visibility would be better, the wind lighter, and, more important, the powder deeper. And, we knew that a trail came through the trees one-half mile or so below that would lead us back to the hut. So, with a few traditional powder hound howls, we pushed off.

The snow was light, the terrain steep. But the narcosis of the deep was creeping in, the nemesis of scuba divers and other depth freaks. So intent was I on making one delirious turn after another that I became intoxicated. I forgot that I hadn't heard John's voice for over a minute. The trail I expected to link up with, which had always been obvious in past trips, was covered over to such an extent that, without realizing it, I skied right over it and down into the trees below. I finally pulled in on the reins of my runaway delirium when I became aware of a sudden, dramatic steepness in the slope.

What a fantastic run, I thought as I watched the forest above for John to slice his way through.

I did my usual yodel. Only silence returned. Knowing how the forest mutes sound, I kept yodeling. After several minutes I concluded he must be below me, waiting at the trail. At least from that vantage point, I would be able to see him if he came out of the trees to my left or right. After all, it was our designated stopping point. So I proceeded down.

Once more I was enraptured by the steep and deep. But suddenly I was brought to full red alert. The terrifying sound of tons of settling snow pierced through my body. Anyone who has witnessed an avalanche, or been in an avalanche, knows the feeling. Absolute vulnerability penetrates your being as the earth

23

seems to drop from under you. The snow may only be "set-tling" a few inches, but it feels as if the whole foundation of your life is giving way in one loud "thump." But I was blessed. I felt only the settling. The feared "slide" of tons of snow down the mountain didn't occur.

My primal survival genes were activated. I looked about. Where the heck was I? What I thought was a great run down to a well-marked trail now felt like an emergency phone call jolt-ing me awake in the middle of the night. I shouted. I listened. Nothing. How could reality change so swiftly? I looked down into a steep narrow valley far below. I looked up. No sign of John. Traversing left or right simply moved me more along the side of the steep valley, possibly triggering an avalanche. How did that trail disappear? Had the snow fallen that much to cover the trail? It couldn't still be below me, could it? Had I just been unconscious, unaware? Was this the trickster side of God showing up in life to test me again? Was this some karmic debt that I had to pay for past sins? Or was I simply dumb, cold, and lost?

Okay. Let's calmly examine the situation. I'm alone at ten thousand feet. I have left my survival gear in the hut. I can't find my ski buddy. It's getting dark. It's snowing, I've missed the trail, I'm stuck on the side of a steep canyon, and I'm dressed for a summer barbecue. *Hey, no problem.*

I'll simply put the skins back on and hike back up my tracks to the missed road. The snow was a couple of feet deep, so it would be fairly heavy trail-breaking, but I should be at the road by dark. I took off one ski and stuck the tail in the snow. Leaving the tip straight up in the air, I pulled the skins from my wind-breaker. They were stiff and frozen. I pulled them apart and placed the loop of one of them over the tip of my ski. I pressed the skin to the bottom of the ski, expecting the glue to adhere as usual. But each time I pressed down, the skin fell loosely away from the ski, like trying to reseal an envelope after you forgot to enclose the check. I nervously tried the other skin. Same result. *Problem.*

More hollers to John. Hollers, not yodels. No answers. I looked to the heavens with that pleading kind of expression, that mixture of anger and helplessness that lack of control brings. But heaven answered only with cold snow and biting wind. The duct tape that could have secured my skins was in my backpack. Everything that I needed to survive out here was in my backpack, sitting only a few feet away from the fireplace in my cozy hut. The duct tape was, no doubt, warm, dry, and secure. The image made me laugh as I hurriedly placed my skis back on, thinking that I was going to be one tired lad by the time I sidestepped up the mountain. Then I realized to my horror that the snow was so deep, and the terrain so steep, that sidestepping was next to impossible. Plus I was wearing telemark skis in which the heel piece was not locked down. With each step, the tail of the ski dangled down into the heavy snow, making it impossible to lift my skis.

Maybe if I took my skis off I could use them as "rafts" to support myself in the heavy snow and scratch and crawl my way up the mountain. *Again, no problem.*

After ten minutes of exhausting work, I had moved only ten feet. Let's see . . . that comes out to one foot per minute. At that rate, I'd be back in the cabin about June 3. I sat in the snow, physically and mentally depleted. The perspiration from my physical effort began to freeze on my skin. Darkness was outracing the light. I can't go down. I can't go up. I'm stuck. I'm cold. I'm scared. Hypothermia would be setting in shortly. *Problem.*

I looked around for possible snow cave location. If I could burrow in deep enough, maybe I could survive the night. It would probably get down to zero outside, but snow is an excellent insulator. I had built snow caves off of cornices before, but there was no cornice here, and the snow was so light it kept falling back as I tried digging. Would the exertion of attempted

25

cave-building increase my chance of hypothermia? Could I really trust myself to not sleep, knowing that sleep can be the kiss of death in the cold?

Then it occurred to me. In all of the physical and mental activity and anguish, I had forgotten to come back to center. My life is about this skill and training; my profession of working with organizations and the general public is based on it. And here I was not using it when I most needed it. Instead of continuing my frantic searching for a way out, my angry and demanding pleading to the heavens for a lifeline, my fearful mind rerunning death scenes and previewing newspaper headlines, and grieving friends and relatives, I sat upright in the snow, with my back against a tree. I began to breathe deep and full, to regain my center. With each inhalation, I visualized calmness and warmth entering each cell from my feet up to the top of my head. With each exhalation, I breathed out awareness and connection to the environment around me.

As I did so, I began to relax, and to turn to God in an open, receptive way, listening for an answer. After a couple of minutes of this profound centered silence, the barely audible answer echoed through the forest and my soul. It was a distant sound, one which I never would have heard in my noisy mental and physical state. I became more centered. I heard it again. It was very faint. It was John's voice. I shouted, but this time in the direction of the sound. I did so from center with real intention of my energy carrying all the way to John. On the third shout I knew that I had made a connection. His voice became less frantic and more directed.

Thank you, God. Once more I had learned the power of letting go, of coming to center to calm the wild winds of my fearful mind, and of listening from a deeper place. The sweetness of life returned ever more fragrant and vital. To breathe, to open up my awareness, to be grateful for life. Can anything be more precious?

As my buddy John emerged from the trees with a smile, he could have easily been an angel. He was definitely mine. My angel with duct tape. . . .

A wintry gust
Disappears amid the bamboos
And subsides to a calm.

—BASHO

DISCOVER YOUR CENTER

You don't have to wait for a crisis like a snowstorm to experience the power of center. As a matter of fact, I wouldn't recommend it. The truth is that you have been centered hundreds of times in your life. It could have been anytime that you were doing something that you truly love, like when you were playing a game as a child, or joyfully involved in a creative project in business or school, a sporting event, a relationship, etc. Remember one of those times in detail, as vividly as you can. What colors, images, sounds, feelings were present?

As you recall any one of those experiences, you will notice there was a heightened sense of awareness and a deepening connection with everything around you. It was a time in which you experienced effortlessness, time seemed to stop, with hours passing like minutes, your feelings and actions flowing spontaneously with the world around you. You've had entire days when you were centered, "in the zone," got every green light on the way to work, thought of a person and they called, wanted food and someone walked by and offered you a snack. Even now as you relive the past experience, you will experience center.

Choosing to be centered will enable you to access a physiology of optimum balance and power and provide a keen focus, resulting

27

9

in being able to perform at your highest level and to live life with passion. Confidence and positive energy will emanate whether you're talking about sensitive issues with your spouse doing homework or chores, or facing anything that you fear, resent, or resist.

Here is a centering exercise to validate and verify a kinesthetic sense of center, one that you can return to very quickly, no matter what your situation—stuck in traffic, relationship crisis, the "big" meeting, or an exam:

• Have a partner stand easily and naturally, with his feet approximately shoulder-width apart.

• Stand beside him, facing in the same direction, so that he feels you are there to support him, not challenge him.

• Reach over and place the fingertips of one hand very lightly just above the center of your partner's chest.

• Very slowly and smoothly increase the pressure on that point, as if you were going to push him directly back. Do so smoothly, with no jerky or sudden motion. Have your partner stand naturally and not try to physically resist this pressure.

• Your partner soon will begin to wobble. Notice how little pressure it took for this to occur.

• Keeping your fingertips in the same position on his chest, ask your partner to concentrate on his center—the physical center of his body—which, in a standing position, is located roughly a couple of inches below the navel. Having him touch that area with his finger will help him to focus his mind on the location.

• Slowly increase the pressure again, gently so as not to distract his thoughts away from his center. It may be helpful to tell him to take any feeling of pressure on the chest down to his center, to actually feel it "from his center."

• As you slowly increase the pressure on his chest, you will find that there is remarkably more stability, gained simply by your partner's becoming more aware of his natural center.

• Now reverse roles and have the partner test you. Always do the centering exercise slowly and consciously, regardless of which role you are playing.

As you relive a peak experience from the past vividly, using all your senses, you can use the centering test again to verify the fact that centering and peak performance are intimately connected. Centering is a natural state that you can choose at any time and strengthen with practice. Each person will experience center differently, as each has his or her own way of remembering or interpreting any event. Some of us are more visual, so centering will be more of a picture. Those who are more kinesthetic will experience centering as a feeling, and others who are predominantly auditory will relate to centering as a vibratory sensation. Or centering may be an overlapping of all three sensations.

The more "cues" you develop to center, the better. I'm not asking you to walk around all day with your finger below your navel. Simply take a moment to recapture your experience—whether visual, auditory, kinesthetic, or all three—periodically throughout the day, and then go about whatever you are doing. Centering doesn't take time; it takes intention.

Centering is not an actual physical point or position. A scientist would describe any object's center of gravity as an infinitely small point or fulcrum upon which that object can be brought into equilibrium or balance. If someone did an in-depth vector analysis of you or a building, they could discover a point upon which either could be balanced. But, by definition, you could continue to divide that point in half until you recognize that there is actually no fixed point. And besides, if you are in dynamic movement in relationship to other forces, like what a ski racer experiences, center will continually shift to maintain dynamic balance.

Thank goodness, you don't have to figure out your center's exact location to develop this skill (otherwise, the only skiers would be physicists). Simply relax and put your awareness where your deepest natural breathing originates—approximately $1\frac{1}{2}$ inches below your navel. Balance will be restored, regardless of your position or movement, without your trying to figure it out.

With practice, you will begin to access center easily in many ways—whether elicited by an image, feeling, sound, or thought. Tiger Woods may become centered by touching a golf club; Bach might have done the same every time he heard great music. With practice you will discover that centering can happen everywhere, even in a medical emergency, or when confronted by anger or fear.

Remember, centering is a dynamic, living quality, not a held feeling. Life happens powerfully as a flow, not a holding on. In the exercise, if a person was pushed too hard, a truly centered individual would not tighten up and fall backward—but instead would step back smoothly with the pressure.

Anytime you choose a centered state, your actions will be more effective and more focused. Remember, however, that the purpose is not to forcefully and continuously think about center while in activity. Instead, it is simply to recapture that quality of feeling (which may only take seconds or less) and then focus on whatever it is you are doing, whether it is pushing off on a steep mogul run, lining up a putt on the eighteenth hole, or writing a report. Let your breathing be deep and full, shake loose any tension in the muscles, and trust that as we tune into center, appropriate actions result naturally without effort.

Coloring Outside the Lines

There is no true path without center.
With center the mind, body, and spirit merge—
Passion and commitment unleash
A force that cannot be contained.

Being lost in a snowstorm was a significant learning experience. But how soon we forget those precious moments of center in the chaos of our lives—the phone calls, the latest body ache, the need to defend our position on every topic in the known universe. What we need, of course, are more learning experiences, forcing us to color *outside* the lines.

Have you noticed that most of the time we react in the same old predictable way to those irritating things in our life—an uncooperative child or parent, a coworker's decision, a friend's broken commitment, or most tragically, a missed three-foot putt? We are on automatic, living each new day from the past, reacting in the same old predictable ways of thinking, feeling, and behaving. We can accomplish almost anything through conscious practice, whether it's obtaining a fifth-degree black belt in aikido or playing Beethoven on the piano. It stands to reason that you can also get your fifth-degree black belt in anger or depression if you practice enough. And many have. We become so unconsciously competent in reproducing the same old unhealthy patterns of behavior, that the rut deepens, every day's the same old day, same old people, same old attitude. We often need a significant event to jar us out of painting by the numbers, awakening us to the magic of coloring outside the lines, to see the world new and fresh each day.

One day I received a call from two community-minded businessmen from Atlanta, Charlie Barton and George Johnson, asking if I would be willing to do something "very different." Well, "very different" sounded intriguing, so I said yes.

They offered me a unique opportunity to do a presentation in Atlanta for eight hundred alienated kids, mostly inner-city, who had quit or been thrown out of high school. Having taught in both public and private schools, I recognized the situation as every teacher's nightmare. Eight hundred teenagers, each a kindred spirit of every kid who had ever failed, or terrorized a classroom, or raised such havoc that they were expelled.

As the students moved into the gym at Emory University, my adrenaline level was rising. With pounds of chains clanging, black leather creaking, and cynical eyes checking me out, they let me know that the average lecture wasn't going to cut it. I'd better have something good to offer, or they'd quickly put an end to any motivation I might have for similar youth work in the future. If I could offer them something that was relevant to their lives in the streets, they'd be committed to get it. If not, they'd be gone. They were not into philosophy, they were into survival.

These were kids that school and society had labeled failures. In my past experiences as a teacher, it was always frustrating that the kids believed and had reluctantly accepted the label, and felt anger and rebellion their only recourse. I considered others that schools had labeled as failures, like Edison, Einstein, Buckminster Fuller, Winston Churchill, to name a few. I wondered if these kids in Atlanta were aware that they were in such classy company?

If cultural diversity creates attention, I certainly had their interest. There I was standing on a twenty-by-twenty-foot mat wearing my traditional aikido gi and hakama (a long black pleated skirt, traditional for teachers of aikido). Their first glimpse of a blue-eyed, blond-haired white guy dressed like a Japanese samurai, standing on a gym floor somewhere in Georgia, let them know that they were in for something different.

I got to the basics of survival right away. They already knew that to make it on the streets they had to be gutsy, tough, and street-smart. I suggested that to do that you had to know something about true strength and power, and calmness under pressure, and that I was going to focus on precisely those skills. Skills that could help them on the streets right now, *today*. I explained that those skills required a mind and a body that worked together—an integrated mind-body state.

I began an aikido demonstration and sixteen hundred skeptical eyes suddenly saw a different way of dealing with conflict. As my assistant attempted attack after attack, only to end up on the ground, they realized they weren't witnessing the typical street image of holding a position and fighting, or giving up and getting torn apart, or freezing into submission. Instead, they saw constant flow and movement, the attacker's fist or foot missing its mark and my utilizing the subsequent lack of balance and energy to neutralize and control the would-be assailant. They witnessed a demonstration of power and resolution with neither side being harmed.

The art of aikido presented tantalizing concepts for kids grounded in street violence. And yet as captivating as the demonstration was, I had the sense that many might see my assistant as a setup "patsy" and that this demonstration had

33

probably been put on hundreds of times. Knowing this, I asked for a volunteer from the audience.

The reaction was not like that at your normal high school assembly, with at most only a football player or some reluctant kid pushed by his buddies coming forward. At least a full 10 percent of these kids wanted their shots at me. With cheers and shouts a dozen of them clanged toward the mats sporting everything from welding goggles to motorcycle boots. I knew I had to make a choice quickly. I pointed at a big strong-looking guy (6'2", 200 lbs.) who also had a gentle face. I may be foolish at times, but no fool. I knew this guy wasn't out for blood because he had come in earlier with a friend and I had worked with him a bit.

When he came onto the mat, I could feel the excitement of the crowd growing. This situation would either win interest in my work—or lose it completely. He was hesitant about what to do. Which was nice. He was letting me dictate the action. I asked him to throw a punch, slapping my stomach and hoping he would use that as an intended target. Sure enough, he threw a punch at the exact area. I pivoted from my center alongside of his extended arm with my hand, sliding easily down his arm to his fist, leading him even more off center than the missed, punch had left him. With a whirling movement of my entire body, as if I were the center and he the rock whirling on the end of a string, I led him into a wrist technique that caused him to fall onto the mat unable to move. The oohs and aahs of the crowd said it all. Here was *something worthwhile.* When the smoke cleared and I had subdued a variety of the young man's kicks and punches, the audience was fully present and ready to learn.

There is nothing quite like committed students. These kids now wanted to know how they could handle the attacks in their lives, whether physical, mental, or social. They began to consider my words. Was it possible to disagree without being disagreeable? Could they resolve differences so that people were honored not abused? Could they get centered anytime and be able to generate power from within and be calm under pressure? You could see their minds spinning. These so called "misfits" and "problem kids" were as attentive and focused on learning as any participants I had ever seen in any school or adult workshop. They were coloring outside the lines.

Instead of leaving immediately after the program ended, these kids gathered around with real questions about tough problems. They were streetwise and street-tough. They didn't see life through rose-colored glasses. To them life was stressful and dangerous, and anything perceived as helpful in negotiating their troubled waters was like a life raft to the shipwrecked. From behind their sunglasses and leather, their essences shined through. They were courageous, eager, and special. I was inspired.

"How can I learn this stuff, man?" asked a short, muscular African-American kid who introduced himself as T.J.

Good question. I was only in town for one day, just an afternoon's entertainment, a brief interlude from their normal life. I knew that what I had to teach wasn't in the standard curriculum either, in his classroom or his local hangout. It wasn't possible to take this kid with me.

I looked at T.J. and took a deep breath from center.

"I'm glad you asked, T.J. Let's start by getting centered again." I moved over so that I was standing alongside him.

T.J. stood relaxed with feet about shoulder-width apart. He placed his hands briefly on his physical center, which he now knew to be about one and a half inches below the navel, and breathed deeply from that area. He focused fully on his center. I reached over and put my hand very lightly just above the middle of his chest. I slowly and gradually increased the pressure on that point, as if I were going to push him directly back. He brought the pressure into his center without resisting against it. He was like a tree. He was strong and stable. (This centering exercise is described in detail on page 28.)

"Good, T.J.! Remember the feeling. Capture that feeling of center so that you can come back to it anytime you choose."

I released the pressure of my hand on his chest.

"Now, think of something that you don't like, a problem or situation that didn't turn out so well. Reexperience that moment in as much detail as possible." As he did, his face hardened, his shoulders sagged, and his energy left him. I tested again. This time he wobbled easily.

"Now, T.J., think of something that you really love to do. And think of a time when you were doing it really well. It doesn't have to be something difficult, it might be just riding a bike, or reading, or creating something, or playing a sport. Anything will do, as long as it was something in which you were performing great or feeling great."

As his mind fully relived it, his body followed. Posture became more erect, his face was relaxed and alert, energy was flowing. I tested again. No wobble. He was stable and powerful, his body energized but not rigid.

"Excellent!" I repeated the process again, going back and forth between the centered and uncentered state, moments in his life that were exceptional and those in which he experienced a series of failures.

"T.J., you went back and forth between wobbling to incredible stability. And yet you were standing in the same position, and I tested the same each time. What changed?"

T.J.'s eyes lit up as if he had just discovered a gold mine.

"Just my mind, man. Just my mind. I just changed what I was thinking about. This is beautiful. I can use this!"

He had gained a real sense of his personal power. He knew that choosing to be centered by focusing on what's working or what could work was a valuable skill that didn't require anything but his moment-by-moment choice.

"T.J., are there things in your life that you would love to do and you know you would be good at if you stayed with them?"

"No doubt. No doubt at all!" T.J. was pumped. He was coloring outside his lines.

Now I was pumped. When you catch a kid with his eyes lit up, you want him to capture that moment so fully that those moments extend out into the rest of his life. So he understands that *he* was doing it, that it wasn't being done *to* him.

A small crowd was gathering around T.J. and me. They were just as turned on as we were. As I glanced from face to face, I saw beyond the labels that they had been given or had taken on themselves. What I saw was a specialness that wanted to be released. As difficult as their lives may have been, they were still looking to find some meaning in their lives, to learn to be successes in their neighborhoods.

And maybe deep down at least some of these kids wanted to share that specialness with others, to add value to their world, and in return to be acknowledged and respected. And maybe, just maybe, centering could help them acknowledge themselves when no one else would.

They began to practice the centering exercise that I had done with T.J. The negative labels began to peel off their brains. Their centered experiences reflected the untapped potential in each of them: "I was fixing my car." "I was taking over top-spot in my gang." "I was jammin' on the drums." "I was throwing some smooth moves in a big game."

Their responses reflected aptitudes that their classroom experiences had never nurtured. They might have an aptitude for the mechanical, musical, athletic, visual, or relational rather than the more traditional three R's. What about an aptitude for leadership (why are those gang leaders so effective?), in entrepreneurship, or in working with animals or nature? If we could nurture their specialness, then their self-esteem and confidence would grow. From a strong base of centered confidence they would expand their learning to other necessary skills and be able to effectively apply their gifts positively in their communities where their enthusiasm will make them natural teachers and models for others. As Lee Iacocca, former chairman and CEO of Chrysler put it, "In a completely rational society, the best of us would be teachers and the rest of us would have to settle for something else."

T.J. held out his hand, and gestured with the other.

"Hey, man, thanks for the day."

He glanced at the other kids and then back to me.

"I don't know about those dudes, but I'm going to practice this stuff."

That made my day. I shook his hand.

"Thanks, T.J., for the gift you've given me."

As I looked into T.J.'s dark brown eyes, I knew that he had to color *far* outside his lines in order to *make* it in society's terms. But what exactly was "making it"?

I thought of my fourteen-year-old son Eri. He had always done well in school—straight A's, athletic, popular, the whole ball of American wax. I am quite proud of that. Yet, without the wisdom of perspective and vision, "credentials" can lead to the need to be perfect in everything, the need to please everybody. They can be a fast track to many medals but a lousy life.

And that's why, after returning from Atlanta, one evening over tacos, I suggested to Eri that he quit school for a year and travel around the world and work with me.

"Let's go live somewhere radically different with no preconceived plans, and see what happens."

And after a few more days of deliberation (far more than I would have taken when I was fourteen) he said in a rock-solid way, "Okay, Dad."

*Ask yourself, and yourself alone, one question. Does this path have
a heart? All paths are the same; they lead nowhere. They are paths
going through the bush or into the brush. . . . Does this path have a
heart? If it does, the path is good; if it doesn't, it is of no use.*
                                        —Don Juan (Carlos Castaneda)

GROW YOUR CENTER

Life is change. And change is asking us to color outside the lines.
T.J., if only for a moment, saw a way out of the boundaries that
were limiting him. Events that shake up our beliefs and perspectives happen to each of us, but too often we miss the opportunity to
step outside the rigid lines of our thinking. We resist change
because we view the situation as a threat to our security, and react
by clinging to our old positions and beliefs. And yet, when we
resist, we lose energy. When we choose to move forward, we gain
energy.

Whenever you find yourself in a difficult or stressful situation,
returning to a centered state is a good first step. Our usual reac-
tions are to fight, flee, or freeze. The martial art of aikido offers
another alternative—**flow**—which translates readily into daily life
applications. When conflict occurs, aikido teaches us to flow by
embodying these principles:

• *Acknowledge.* Be aware that you have a conflict and what
your feelings are about that conflict. Appreciate the other side's
feelings and viewpoint without labeling them or judging them good
or bad.

• *Accept.* Show the other side that you want to work out a solution. Take responsibility for the fact that you are also part of the
conflict and that all sides are in this together.

• *Adapt.* Be willing to change and be open to new ideas. Be able
to consider a wide range of solutions without excessive judgment.

It takes center to live these principles. When stress occurs, pause, breathe deeply from center, and regain what you recognize as a centered state. The stronger your ability to distinguish between centered and uncentered (a skill that comes with practice), the easier it becomes for you to choose a centered state.

Another aikido exercise that inspired T.J. and the students was the unbendable arm exercise. This demonstrated to them that true power is energy flowing freely to a purpose. It contradicts more traditional perceptions of strength as toughness and rigidity. You can try it yourself.

Stand with a partner of equal or greater physical strength and have him try to bend your arm at the elbow by pulling down on your biceps with one hand and pushing your wrist up with the other, applying a constantly increasing pressure, not a jerky motion. Inevitably, if you are conditioned like the great majority of people on the planet today, you will clench your fist, grit your teeth, and tense up your whole arm, prepared to resist his force by using force directly against him. By applying the proper leverage, he will be able to bend your arm after a few moments. If he cannot, you can still get a sense of how much effort it took to keep him from bending it.

Now imagine your center as an infinite reservoir of water with your arm as a fire hose and your fingers as the nozzle.

First, put no water in the hose (that is, let your arm go limp) and have your partner attempt to bend it. No problem.

Then, as you did in the try-to-be-strong-through-tension example, put "ice" in the hose, as if it had been left outside in subfreezing weather, and have your partner try to bend it again. With enough pressure, the ice will "break" and your arm will suddenly bend.

Finally, turn on that infinite supply of water from your center and allow it to spray out your finger-nozzle. Let your fingers wave easily back and forth to ensure that your muscles don't tense up inadvertently. Relax your shoulder and visualize the stream of water flowing out from the center, up through your body, and out through your shoulder and arm. Keep your elbow slightly bent, not locked. Opening up your senses and imagination, *see, feel,* and *hear* the water spraying out from your extended fingers as far as you can conceptualize—through walls, trees, mountains, people. Your power will increase even more if you visualize the water/energy flowing strongly toward something meaningful to you, that is, a clear purpose such as a child or friend in need of your support. Your partner will find your arm unbendable. Notice, in this more integrated state of mind and body, how much more relaxed and aware you are.

Just as a fully turned-on fire hose is pliable, yet unbendable and unbreakable, your arm will stay soft to the touch, giving a little but not breaking down from the external pressure. Your arm is now connected to your own center and to the world through flowing energy. To bend it, your partner has to contend not with a few muscle fibers but with an unlimited river of energy.

Use those moments when you are standing in line or driving to work to check out your centeredness and let your energy expand. Develop "anchors" or signals to center during daily occurrences in your life—e.g., walking through your office door, turning on your computer, washing your hands.

Notice the daily events that are likely to push you off center or tend to make you shut down. Create supports to help you stay centered in these situations. For example, let's say you were a customer service representative and you found yourself vulnerable to irate customer phone calls. Use the first ring of the telephone as an opportunity to breathe deeply from the abdomen and to center on your highest ability to add value to the caller. In addition (it helps if no one is looking), you might bow slightly to the phone in gratitude for the opportunity to center and then pick it up on the second or third ring, all with the concentration of a master performing a tea ceremony.

You can also practice centering by imagining a future activity

41

and capturing that centered state. For example, imagine yourself on the eighteenth hole of a golf course about to make a critical putt that will complete the best game of your life. As you get ready to putt, imagine what is going on inside you—quiet thoughts, calmness, control, an almost eerie awareness of your surroundings, everything happening in slow motion. Visualize the ball falling neatly into the cup. Hear that rattling sound as it hits the bottom. Feel a sense of warmth and relaxation. Positive imaging. Imaging the future, using all the senses, is a great way to enter a centered state.

Letting Go

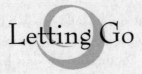

To center is to relax the tight fist of clinging.
Into the open hand falls freedom.

The orange-clad monk smiled at our blond hair.

"From where you come?" he asked.

I wondered if he could understand how far away the Rocky Mountains actually were from this Buddhist temple in southern Thailand, and yet how much at home I really felt.

"America?" he beamed, and then pointed at himself: "I student of English!"

He handed me a book in English on Buddha's four noble truths. As I opened it, my eyes came to rest on a page dealing with the origin of suffering. Buddha says that the root of all suffering stems from attachment—attachment to ourselves, to our possessions, to our activities, to our opinions.

I looked at my teenage son, Eri. Here we were on our father-and-son journey to new places and new ideas, exploring the world with all our senses, finding real sights and sounds, smells and tastes—things you can't get through textbooks and television. We were taking a year off from what we thought was our life, to discover what else it could be. Two boys, one in his forties and the other fourteen, both celebrating a rite of passage of sorts, wandering in Southeast Asia—our backpacks filled with camera, clothing, and assorted garbage.

Reading the wisdom of Buddha's words, Eri and I found ourselves nodding in agreement with the principle of nonattachment. I stared at the shaven-headed monk. He was radiant.

"What do you do at the monastery?"

"I sit here," he smiled, as if bewildered by such a question. "I sleep there," motioning to the small hut behind him. "I eat there," indicating the kitchen across the temple yard. "I study. I greet people who come by. Would you like some tea?"

This man seemed to have something special going for him. And it surely didn't come from his possessions—orange tunic and sandals, a few books, and a mattress and blanket. Not a computer game in sight. No, he wore his happiness inside out. It came through his eyes, through his smile, from somewhere deep inside.

I was captivated.

"How long have you been here?"

"Ten years," he said as naturally as we would say "a few hours."

"When did you become a monk?"

"When I was thirteen," he said, smiling at Eri.

Eri and I glanced at each other, stunned. When he was a year younger than Eri was now, this man had made such a momentous choice, a definite rite of passage alien to an average American teenager—or to his father, for that matter.

We felt good just sitting there; the three of us.

I reflected on attachment.

Life does seem to get easier when I let go a bit. There are the little things like giving away old clothes or tossing out old files after years of pack-ratting. Then there are the big things, like letting go of an unworkable relationship or a job that made money but no sense.

I know the difficulty of most pack rats like myself. You just never know when that magazine article on healing headaches by placing cold cucumber slices on your forehead will come in handy or when that disgusting shirt will be perfect for some costume party. And yet, after the pain of tossing it into the recycling bin, a feeling of freedom arises. With practice, we can remember that feeling, and go on a roll—like letting go of the anger we feel in rush-hour traffic, or the defensiveness we feel when someone makes a suggestion, and, eventually, the attachment to the ego, our youth, even (gulp) our physical health. There is simply a greater sense of peace after letting go of the clinging.

After a deeply peaceful afternoon it was time to bid good-bye to our new friend. After taking a few pictures, Eri and I climbed into our beat-up old open Jeep that we had rented for a few dollars a day. We waved to the smiling monk one last time. As I turned a corner to go out the gate, our camera began to slide off the dashboard.

"Stop!" Eri shouted.

Too late. We watched it crash on the ground behind us. Eri jumped out and returned, dangling from his fingers what was left of our expensive Nikon camera, now better suited for duty as a paperweight. A flash of anger arose in both of us as we looked for some way to justify this, someone to accuse.

"I can't believe you left it on the dashboard!" was roaring out of my mouth precisely as "Why'd you turn so fast!" was flashing out of Eri's. Out of our peripheral vision we caught the image of the monk still beaming and waving at us with his heart wide open. It framed the absurdity of the moment. We stopped in mid-rage. Instantly, we knew. The first test of Buddha's principle of nonattachment had occurred within minutes of learning it.

An embarrassed smile formed on Eri's face. Our tantrums were cut short.

Thus began our new discipline of letting go. We drove down the road. Peaceful and wise. For a few minutes. And then one of us would be angry about the camera again. But the other would remind him of our new practice.

"No clinging, Dad, just breathe and get centered. Like you always teach."

Was I going to have to put up with this the entire trip?

But each time we noticed the angry feeling beginning to rise, so did the monk's smile, Buddha's words, and an old mindfulness prayer:

> *Breathing in, I calm body and mind.*
> *Breathing out, I smile.*
> *Dwelling in the present moment,*
> *I know this is the only moment.*

The test for letting go was just beginning. Somehow I think God knew we were just novices and that more training was needed. Each day it was something else—misplaced keys, passport, scuba mask, and more. It kept the pressure on to really let go. After a couple of arduous weeks we thought we had it made, the principle of letting go firmly established. So much so, we even purchased a new camera. Ah, yes, we had paid our dues, nothing could hook us now. Let go, and let God. And ready to take some good pictures!

46

9

It was late afternoon some days later on the tenth hole of a jungle golf course. Eri and I are both avid golfers. If there is one other constant in life, besides change, it is that golf can be played *anywhere,* even in the jungles of Southeast Asia. I was about to nail my approach shot to the green when a monkey came out of the jungle behind us and began to cross the fairway. We had never seen a monkey in the wild before (especially the wilds of a golf course), and Eri immediately took out our new camera.

As Eri approached, the animal growled, bared its teeth, and made an ugly swipe with its hand. Eri backed up and froze. Then out of the forest emerged four baby monkeys and what looked like the mother. The threatening gesture must have been to protect the babies. We smiled at this unique sight, something never seen at the famous St. Andrews or Pebble Beach links. Finally, a large male with a full beard, jagged teeth, and a Clint Eastwood squint emerged and slowly began to knuckle his way directly toward us. Despite all my years of martial art training, I suddenly realized I was devoid of aikido techniques for big monkeys. One look at the size of his arms made me thankful that I was holding a five-iron. With each step that he took toward us, we backed away. But he kept coming.

"What do we do, Dad?" Eri asked nervously.

I told Eri, "Judging the lie the monkey has, and the distance to the pin, a five-iron is the club of choice."

Eri grabbed a three-wood. He rarely takes my golf tips.

Laughing, we stayed calm and relaxed, rather enjoying the encounter. The monkey seemed more relaxed too and began to develop an interest in my recently abandoned golf bag. He began touching the clubs and picking up my ball and tossing it, as if to say "I don't play Top-Flites. Do you have any Titleists here?"

I said to Eri, "This will make some great photos."

Just then, at the same moment, all three of us saw the camera on the ground near the golf bag where Eri had left it when he picked up the three-wood. The monkey eyed the camera carefully.

So much for my practice of letting go. I had a massive recurrence of *the clings* as I saw this macho primate approach *my* camera. So much for my unattached attitude. All fear vanished. I

47

9

stepped forward to claim what was rightfully mine. *My stuff!* "Hey, don't even think about it, you big . . ." But I was frozen in my tracks by one fixed make-my-day glare. So much for my power of intention.

The monkey reached down and swooped up the camera. The *new* camera. *My brand-new camera!*

I tried mental telepathy.

"That's *my* camera, not *your* camera," I lasered into his hairy skull.

So much for mental telepathy. He nonchalantly removed the case, tossed it over his shoulder, took the camera, and held it up to his eye.

Now I know this sounds like too much artistic license, and I'm sure if I didn't have a witness to corroborate the story, I couldn't trust myself with repeating it. But I swear that this monkey, this hairy primate with beady eyes, began to mimic a professional fashion photographer, as if working on the proper angles and lighting.

"Beautiful, beautiful, you two look great, beautiful! Work with me!"

After a minute or so, satisfied and rather pompous, he wrapped the camera strap around his wrist and ambled off into the jungle. The ultimate test for a case of the clings! There, in the approaching darkness, were father and son, with five-iron and three-wood in hand, walking nervously through the jungle in Southeast Asia, following a monkey who had stolen their camera. To what strange karmic past did I owe such a teaching?

Exposing more human inadequacy, the monkey gracefully and swiftly ascended sixty feet up a tree. We agonized as he swung happily from branch to branch, banging our camera along with him.

Mercifully, an idea surfaced.

"Remember the book *Caps for Sale*?" I asked.

48

"Of course," Eri replied, "you read it to me a hundred times when I was little."

It was a children's story about a cap peddler who carried twenty caps in a stack on his head. At lunch, as he sleeps leaning against a tree, nineteen naughty monkeys each steal a cap, put it on, and climb up into the tree. Upon wakening, the peddler explodes in anger. The monkeys mimic everything he does. He waves his arms, they wave theirs. He stomps his feet, they stomp theirs. Finally, in total frustration, he throws down his remaining cap on the ground—and violà! Nineteen caps come flying out of the tree.

The solution was *obvious.* We began to throw clubs, coconuts, rocks, golf balls, and sunglasses to the ground, all with one eye on our hairy friend. He began to study our antics. "We've got him now," I whispered, proudly confident, to Eri, as the monkey looked down at us and back at our camera.

He fingered it intently. Then, in the honored lineage of all the great masters, he opened the battery compartment, removed the two batteries, and in a frivolous gesture tossed them at our feet.

The sun had set. Two boys, one in his forties and the other fourteen, lay laughing on the jungle floor, looking up at a bemused hairy relative. They had been forced to give up a killer case of the clings. Let go, let God. Relax and enjoy. Everything is unfolding perfectly. And, after all, we did get the batteries back.

And as soon as we really let go, what do you think happened? Did we end up getting what we wanted with the monkey tossing down our camera? It would make a nice ending, right? But, the last principle of letting go is that it is not a manipulative technique to control the universe. Bucky Fuller once said, "You did not create this universe and you do not control it." However, if you ever stumble across a monkey somewhere in Southeast Asia carrying a Nikon camera, follow him. It was a good camera.

In my ten-foot bamboo hut
this spring
There is nothing
There is everything.

—SODO

LEARN TO LET GO

The concept "letting go" is enticing. Wouldn't you like to let go of your sense of burden, your stress, your fearful, judgmental, and unhappy thoughts? Wouldn't you like to let go of your need to control things that you have no control over—the weather, another's approval, your past history?

You'd think it would be easy to let go of these because they are so obviously detrimental. But we have gone through a superb training in a mind-set that locks us into suffering unnecessarily. Let's call this mind-set the Perfection Syndrome, which looks good on the surface, yields a measure of success of life, but in the end creates struggle, stress, and emptiness.

Yet, the key to "letting go" is through what could be called the Discovery Process. Kids arrive on this planet with the Discovery Process intact—an innate sense of curiosity, fully ready to participate, and bursting with creativity. Those traits allow them to learn the really difficult tasks like walking and talking. But over time we tend to botch up the natural learning process. We think that we have to be perfect, and in trying to do so, we base our self-esteem on how well we perform or how we compare to a model. We have to perform at a certain level or look like a certain individual or group in order to feel okay. All of this leads to a dominating question, "Am I right or wrong?"

Every conflict starts to be seen as a contest, where being right is the goal, and seeking viable solutions takes a back seat. With your concern about being right, a fear of failure enters. Self-esteem based upon performance or a model leaves you focused on the outer world, and appearances. You begin to think that you're alone in the middle of the Coliseum of Life, with the whole world as spectators holding up score cards. You become so focused on not failing that you become hesitant and resist stepping out fully into life.

Imagine if you had to relearn to walk. Each stumble and fall would be labeled as a failure. And, how many of those failures would it take before you refused to practice in front of others, or eventually at all? Contrast that to one-year-olds learning to walk. What is their expression when they are falling, which we perfection-obsessed adults would label as failing? Is it not joyful awareness? And, what happens right after the act of falling? Every kid, every culture? They look up, with wide-open enthusiasm and a natural desire to proceed. Their criteria for self-esteem is not based on a performance standard or someone's approval. It is simply the joy of learning and growing.

The universe is always changing. But in the Perfection Syndrome, you tend to swim upstream against change, trying to control your environment instead of working with it, all to avoid the possibility of failure. The need to control brings a harsh, judging attitude about things. You end up, no matter how successful your life looks on the trophy shelf, stressed out and burned out.

Peak performance occurs when you are able to reach out and discover, using the natural essence of self—creativity, inquiry, and aliveness. When you operate from these qualities, rather than perfection, the questions that you ask are not whether you are right or wrong but "What can I learn? What am I feeling? What value am I adding?" These questions lead you not to be concerned about failure but to be fascinated with the outcomes of your actions. And that fascination gives birth to the key to peak performance—awareness. Through awareness you make adjustments naturally. That's how kids learn to walk and talk so easily!

When you come from awareness, you can be spontaneous. You are secure in yourself, in your deep connection with the universe. Therefore, you can step out in life, asking "How can I contribute? How can I make a difference?"

As you define yourself not so much by how "perfect" you are, but instead by your desire to learn and to fully participate in life, you begin to appreciate yourself and others. It is the key to good, powerful teams. It is the place where you build trust. You are able to see beyond the negativity of judgment and naturally assume the positive potentiality of humans. This deep place of center, of discovery, allows you to enter the realm of play—meaning full joy and participation in whatever you are doing. That place allows you to add value, no matter what the activity—washing dishes or running a company. You do not need entitlement or someone's approval to add value—only a commitment to learn and to serve others.

When you are in a conflict, first get centered and breathe deeply. This will allow you to suspend the knee-jerk reaction of seeing the conflict as a contest. This "conflict equals contest" mentality directs us to thinking, What do I need to do or say to be right? You will unconsciously pull the other person into his own competitive nature and the war begins. Instead, ask the more powerful question, What do I need to learn? Your primary desire to learn about the other side and to be open to new ideas should not be construed as admitting that the other side is right or that you're shrinking in the face of opposition. Instead, by being open to discovery, you are taking a courageous step toward resolution.

This opens the door for the adversarial nature of the relationship to shift into a partnership, inviting dialogue toward creative solutions. The key is letting go of what you think you know. How much of all there is to know in the universe do you know? Since we all know that the percentage is infinitesimally small, why spend so much time and energy trying to be right about so little?

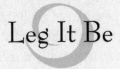Leg It Be

To center is to embrace the tiger of our fear
and return to the mountain of our higher self—
connected, joyous, and aware.
"Embrace Tiger, Return to Mountain."

Modern science teaches that evolution and transformation can arise out of chaos. Chemist Ilya Prigogine, a Nobel laureate, shook the scientific world with his theories on disequilibrium.

> *When a molecule's implicate (existing) order starts to fall apart, the entity faces a moment of choice, the 'bifurcation point.' It can either go out of existence, or reorganize itself at a higher level to accommodate the new variables.*

This is good stuff to chew on. Quite a choice we have. Either change or die. You'd think humans would have no problem making such a decision.

Understanding this chaos theory, it's easy to see why we often need to get lost in order to learn something new. An important step occurs when we are willing to be totally confused—we can get centered, give up trying to control the universe, and enter into the magic realm of discovery.

When I teach the martial art of aikido, I sometimes recognize that my students are having a difficult time with a relatively simple move, primarily because they are trying too hard to get it right. For instance, if I'm working with a student on handling a straight punch to the stomach, I teach a specific pivot or turn, allowing her to move out of the line of the attacking fist but still maintain a connection with the assailant's arm. This circular movement puts her in a more appropriate position from which to neutralize, control, or throw the attacker. However, if she is too mechanically involved in the technique, or fearfully staring at the oncoming fist, her reaction time will be slower than normal, and her movement more clumsy. She has forgotten the flow, the ability of the body to move effortlessly from center. To help center her, I have more than one person attack, one after another in rapid succession and from different angles. At first she is paralyzed by the increase in complexity, but within moments she is forced to let go of the step-by-step mechanics, and her need to control. She spontaneously becomes centered. It's better than getting punched. She begins to move quickly and more efficiently. Her awareness shifts to include a bigger perspective than one little fist, as she must now be aware of multiple attackers (with multiple fists) coming from different directions. She has no choice but to trust her center and continue moving. There is no time to intellectualize and judge her performance. After a few minutes I ask her to go back to a single attacker. Centered, her body flows with ease, far more relaxed than when she first began. Her feet move naturally. Her mind is more present and aware of the whole person, not just a fist. "This technique is not as hard as I thought" is the typical reply.

Chemist Prigogine would have been proud. The student naturally chose to reorganize at a higher level to accommodate new variables. Such a choice has a lot to do with centering, which in turn has to do with trust.

In the previous chapter the teaching of center came from the monk and the monkey. But now Eri and I find ourselves in the mountains of northern Thailand. Our new teacher is the mud. As you will see, that is *not* a metaphor. I'm talking red mud. Wet dirt from hell.

The Golden Triangle is the name of the infamous region that borders Thailand, Burma, and Laos, where the great percentage of the world's heroin and opium trade originates. Lush jungles and beautiful poppy-laden mountain valleys conjure up mixed images of Shangri-la and danger. With the billions of dollars in worldwide narcotics at stake, I knew that my son Eri and I would be easily expendable if we innocently ended up in the wrong place at the wrong time. But the lure of jungle- and mountain-trekking in that exotic part of the world overrode such gangster concerns.

We found ourselves in the picturesque city of northern Thailand, Chiang Mai. This aesthetic city, rich with temples, now appeared to have more motorcycles than people. But as late as 1920, it could only be reached by river or by elephant. It is the gateway to another culture, the mountainous tribal region, inhabited by Sino-Tibetan and Burmese-Tibetan people (called the Montagnard). Along with, of course, the drug lords.

We stayed at one of the numerous inexpensive ($5 a night) "homestays," and began our search for a personal guide for a trek. We had steered clear of the commercial trek services, for fear that we would find ourselves along the well-trodden tourist routes where everyone would, for a tip, play a role à la Disney World instead of revealing their real lives. It was outside our homestay that we met a young Thai who called himself Tak (only because he knew we would have had difficulty pronouncing his real name). He captivated us immediately with his energized smile and oversized white tennis shoes with Mickey Mouse pictures all over them. The man smelled of adventure.

Tak engagingly declared he could provide us with the "best trek with best of everything"—elephant trek to poppy/opium

9

country, sleeping in a remote jungle village, and good home cookin' (his, of course). I thought it would be a good test of his tour-guiding acumen if he first took us shopping for the best deal on a tape recorder. Eri wanted to record our dialogues with different cultures for his new audio journal, since the photo journal idea had been sabotaged by the aforementioned primate (or was it divine?) intervention.

"No worry," smiled Tak. He drove us through clogged traffic like a veteran New York cabdriver, and haggled with a shop-keeper as well as any camel-seller I had seen in Egypt. I knew we had found our man.

The next morning we were ready to go. To our surprise, Tak had also convinced a young couple from France to go along with us. In numbers, I was feeling more confident already. He insisted that we didn't need to bring anything but a daypack, as all would be provided for in the village where we would stay. Had this been a movie, here is where the suspense music would begin.

Driving north, we visited some of the typical tourist spots along the Burma-Thai border before stopping in the mountain town of Chiang Rai. We hung on to Tak's shirt as we weaved and negotiated his way through a crowded, open food market buying things that resembled vegetables and fruit. But the dirt, smell, and steamy clutter of the place neutralized any appetite that Eri and I may have had.

With his pack full, his energizing smile intact, Tak led us off to the banks of the Kok River to rent a long skinny boat called a hang yao. We could most easily access the jungle and mountain villages by river. A sinewy little man with few teeth and fewer words cranked up the small outboard motor, and in a few min-utes we were escaping the stifling heat of the day and the bustling, hustling throngs of the city. Cool breezes from the boat's movement kept us free of bugs. We began to relax into a mystical ride down the twisting narrow little river. From time to time, we were entertained by children bathing, and people doing laundry alongside quaint old villages that we floated by. The vivid colors of the women's clothing enhanced the lush green of the surrounding countryside. With each turn of the river we left more of civilization behind, eventually seeing only a lonely hut or an occasional bird competing for fish with a few men working their nets along the shore. The present floated into the past. The long, skinny hang yao felt strangely familiar, and I imagined that an ancient Siam would have received us warmly, white skin, funny hats, and all.

Within the hour, the sun would be down. Surely we would be stopping soon, as our intention was to spend the night in a remote mountain village. Tak pointed up around the bend. Sure enough, a little cluster of thatched-roof huts and a bamboo pier appeared in the distance. A few children gathered on the banks, wide-eyed and laughing. The boat pulled alongside the rickety pier. We climbed out and without a world the boatman turned around and headed back upstream. I felt my umbilical cord to security had been cut. Some old wrinkled villagers sat on their haunches eyeing the peculiar group of aliens that had just landed.

"So this is the mountain village we're staying in?" I exclaimed, wondering what a mountain village was doing down by the river.

"Oh, no, now we must hike," Tak said through a big smile, pointing past the swampy rice fields toward the jungle-covered hills to the north. "No worry."

It was then that his off-repeated phrase "no worry" began to worry me. The sun was low on the horizon and dropping fast.

The Frenchman Jean-Paul voiced his concern, "Won't it be difficult to see?"

"No worry, I have torch," came the confident reply.

Intuition is a tricky phenomenon. It's like a mosquito looking for a juicy place to land. It's real, it jolts us to attention, but then we

9

try to swat the little pest away, irritated that it is interfering with the logical flow of things. Intuition often flies directly in the face of the rationale of the moment, asking us to shift gears or change direction, which usually means confronting somebody or something, making life more uncomfortable for all concerned. Since our tendency is to shy away from discomfort, we use guilt or the fear of losing someone's approval to swat the annoying feeling out of our path which, by the way, probably leads into a crevasse. Why is it that it's usually after we are picking ourselves up from the bottom that we finally recognize the power of intuition?

Remember those sleepless nights when the drone of a single mosquito haunted you? The high-pitched buzz growing nearer and louder, looking for a juicy runway. *Bzzzzzzzz.*

And, like our intuition, we swat it away.

He's the guide, therefore he *must* know what he's doing, I tell myself. *Bzzzzzzzz.*

Heaven forbid, I don't want to complain and make anybody uncomfortable, I think. *Bzzzzzzzz.*

A half hour later we were wading through ankle-deep mud making our way to the foothills on the other side of the rice paddies.

"*Le trek—c'est impossible!*" grumbled Lisa as she and Jean-Paul held each other up in the gunk.

I looked at Eri, who looked like any fourteen-year-old when asked to do the dishes. I gave him the "This is a great adventure, isn't it" look that all kids immediately recognize as BS, a weak attempt at assuaging my parental guilt from the poorly made decision to be here in the first place.

I could see by the guide's expression that he hadn't expected this much moisture either.

"I've never been on this trek so soon after monsoon," he apologized, nervously surveying his surroundings. "We must keep going."

Why? What horrible thing would happen if we stopped? *Bzzzzzzzz*.

I couldn't help but notice that his permanent smile had ceased to exist.

About an hour later it became evident that the entire trail had been washed out, leaving us a narrow mud trough to wallow through. Darkness had come and it was extremely slippery. After each of us had taken a few spills in the mud, I politely suggested that this would be a good time for our guide to use his "torch," which I of course assumed meant a flashlight.

"No worry." He took off his knapsack and proceeded to rummage inside. To our collective astonishment he emerged with a box of matches. Matches? I looked at Eri. He's kidding, isn't he?

"Don't you have a flashlight?" I queried.

"No worry," he grinned, "I have torch." He began to gather some bark and grasses and sticks together. How ingenious. He's going to make a real old-fashioned torch. Everything is okay now!

Fifteen minutes later he was still trying to light it.

"Too wet," he muttered as each of us searched the heavens, hoping for a miraculous return to daylight. But the moonless sky was pitch-black.

At least nothing else could go wrong.

Then it began to rain. Hard.

Our fearless guide once more dove into his pack. He took out an old shirt and tore it into thin strips and wrapped them around a stick. Next he pulled out his cooking oil, doused the creation, and lit the match. Within a few seconds it ignited and voilà, a torch! A stroke of genius, I thought, having already forgotten the more basic question—how come he didn't have a flashlight? And how come I hadn't brought mine?

Ten minutes later the creative shirt torch went out. Whereupon Tak tied more shirt pieces, used more cooking oil, and trudged on until that torch went out. We stumbled and sludged our way behind him, until many shirts later, Tak dove into his pack and came up empty-handed. He looked up, his eyes fixed on Eri.

Now there's one thing that's sacred to guys everywhere—old T-shirts. No mom or wife worthy of the job would violate the unspoken code and throw one out. But here we were in the jungles of Southeast Asia, doomed. First went Eri's "Flying Dog Brew Pub" T-shirt. Then, sniff, there went my "Oklahoma State Wrestling" shirt. Next went Jean Paul's sweat-stained striped tank top, which I personally was delighted to see go up in smoke. We were at the mercy of a madman, dripping with cooking oil and a lousy sense of direction.

This solemn lineage of torches carried us through the darkness. Our enthusiasm was kindled only by the prospect that Lisa's shirt might be next. But, alas, the cooking oil ran out.

Darkness returned. Images battered at the windmills of my mind—my brand-new headlamp sitting comfortably in our room back in Chiang Mai, right next to my first-aid kit and my Swiss Army knife. I'd religiously carried those jungle essentials everywhere from Honolulu to Bangkok, in airports and bus stations, in all those civilized places where you'd never think of setting up camp. And where are they *now?* I imagine my duct tape from chapter 1 is there too.

That's when the old Sufi saying hit me with real impact: "Trust God, but tie your camel." *bzzzzzz*.

Now the camera and the monkey had given the words "Trust God" real meaning. But without the "tie your camel" corollary, we found ourselves knee-deep in trouble without a light to see our way out. Did it always have to take this much drama to understand the true meaning of those sayings? I couldn't help but shiver over the event that must have befallen the poor Arab lad who had first come up with the camel phrase.

It's fascinating how quickly a fun party can go downhill. Mutinous thoughts had been building a number of shirts earlier. Stumbling around in a swamp had been only disconcerting in the daylight, but with the onslaught of night, it was another story. The shadows elicited all those creepy, crawling images of snakes and leeches, setting off my own mental dialogue. What is under all this water and mud? At least if I could see, I could pick the leeches off or scream if I spotted a slithering movement in the water. I tried to retrieve some solace from Henry David Thoreau.

> *I enter the swamp as a sacred place—*
> *there is the strength, the marrow of Nature.*

But then I remembered I wasn't *in* Massachusetts. Thoreau had very few giant pythons in his pond. All the Hollywood jungle nightmares from Tarzan to Rambo flashed through my cerebral movie screen. I'll never watch *The African Queen* again. I scrutinized Eri. He had trusted me. And probably for the last time, my guilt-ridden brain shot back.

"How ya doin, buddy?" I shouted to him, faking a good time.

"Not bad," came the reply, just as fake.

I noticed by the tonal sharpness of what I had once thought to be a romantic language that our new French friends, Jean-Paul and Lisa, weren't having a lot of fun either.

The stumbling about was exhausting. The falling was terrifying. I would step off a rut (which I later found out to be large animal tracks) and slip to my knees or worse, winding up with mud and microbes in my mouth, scrambling to stand before some reptile could wrap itself around me. It's a funny feeling when mud oozes up your leg in the dark. How can you be sure it's mud, and not something else?

I was in the middle of one of these stumbling splashes when the sound came. We all froze in attention and stared into the darkness.

Our guide whispered, "No move." Not a good sign.

The rumbling and grumbling sound was very close and sounded like it was above our heads. But since our final torch had gone out, I could not be sure where it came from, or what it was, only that it was big. A noise in the dark is always magnified, but this one kept getting louder and closer. Branches were breaking all around us and the snorting seemed only a few feet away. I changed my thinking about big. This thing was breaking *trees*. It was *really* big. Center, stay centered.

"What is it?" Eri whispered.

"Shh," came the guide's reply. "Wild elephant."

Ah, must be even worse than a pet elephant.

Jeez, here I was concerned about leeches and snakes in knee-deep gunk, and we get trampled from above by a nearsighted, ticked-off, or worse, amorous, elephant. A small tree cracked only a few meters above me and to my right. Reflexively, Eri and I grabbed each other in alarm. I expected the myopic monster to come crashing down on us, either by accident or out of discontent (maybe he liked leeches less than I did). But the next major crack of a shrub came a few feet farther away than before, as we realized that he was moving away from us. Thank God, I thought. Now we can focus on the mud and the crawling things again. I made a mental note that, should we survive, I would definitely broaden my study of aikido technique to include not just monkeys but pachyderms.

It's pitch-dark. It's raining hard. We're knee-deep in mud. In my seminars I teach people how to deal effectively with fear, so do you think I was scared? Nah.

I was terrified.

In my workshops I use the acronym F.E.A.R.—for Fantasy Experienced As Real. But, at this point the acronym stood for F—— Everything And Run.

First of all, trekking knee-deep in a swampy water in a Southeast Asian jungle in the pitch-dark put me on shaky mental and physical ground, and the strange, oozing snakelike movements around my legs pulled away any sense of peace. Whenever sounds emerged from the quiet, dark, unknown of the night, we snapped to attention. Fear shadowed our every step.

I needed to start practicing what I teach—to get back to my center, to begin to focus on my breathing, and take one step at a time. The sound of Eri sloshing around behind me gave me added motivation; I had to be fully present if anything should happen. As I focused on my center, my balance improved, my power in stepping through the mud grew, and just as surely my fear level diminished. But the tension of the moment was still there, like a fully stretched rubber band ready to snap.

And when the snap came, I was totally unprepared. It wasn't a scream, or a curse, or a shout at something in the dark. It was a full-blown belly laugh. Tak had tripped over a bush and fallen face down in the swamp. When he emerged, he just sat there with his head peeking out of the mud, laughing. It was utterly contagious. The tension snapped into howls of laughter.

The absurdity of the whole situation—five people falling down in a swamp of pachyderm dung—outweighed the anxiety, if not the elephant. The grand perspective of the whole human predicament that we had chosen to create was vividly exposed, and the cosmic humor accompanying such a state burst through. Now we were all laughing. Somebody would go down, with a splat and a joyful shout, followed by laughter and jokes. You can only get so muddy and so tense before you let go.

Eri, an incurable Beatles buff, found occasion to burst into song:

"When I find myself in times of trouble . . . /Speaking words of wisdom, Let it be."

The snakes, leeches, and other creatures parted like the Red Sea as the maniacal quintet sloshed and sang their way through the muck. Loudest of all sang Tak, his guttural Thai vernacular adding a new dimension to the chorus:

"Leg it be, leg it be, /Speaking words of wisdom, leg it be."

Leg It Be?

And we're a team for the first time! You understand what I'm talking about here? And of course, before we knew it, we rounded a bend and what did we see? The lights of a village in the distance—real torches that stayed lit—nothing was more beautiful to our eyes. Now, we probably would have gotten out of there without the change in attitude. But I know it would have taken a lot longer.

Without a jot of ambition left
I let my nature flow
where it will.
There are ten days of rice
in my bag,
and by the hearth,
a bundle of fire wood.
Who prattles of illusion
or nirvana?
Forgetting the equal dusts of
name and fortune,
listening to the night rain
on the roof of my hut,
I sit at ease
both legs stretched out.

—*RYOKAN*

TURN FEAR INTO POWER

9

When you are paralyzed with fear, you are literally stuck in time. You are worried about a future possibility based on a real (or imagined) past, thus the acronym F.E.A.R.—Fantasy Experienced As Real.

My fear in the swamp could have been based on "I'll be strangled by a snake like I saw in *Ramar of the Jungle*" or "I've heard stories of leeches so big that you have to cut them off with a knife."

When you are in fear, you are trapped in an illusion of time, oscillating between anxiety about something that might happen (the future) and something that you perceived did happen (the past). The best way to deal with fear is to go to the place where fear isn't—the present. When you are in the present with full awareness, fear no longer paralyzes you and you are able to respond appropriately with power and grace be it in an office, your living room, or a swamp. The key is to come to center and into greater awareness of your senses—breathing, seeing, feeling.

As you center, you will have an increased awareness of how your fear is reflected in your body. Breathing deeply, you can gradually relax the areas of your body that are contracted in tension because of your fear. To develop this skill, ask yourself specific kinesthetic questions such as: Where am I carrying this fear—my throat, stomach, neck, knees? Analyze it—specifically, how big is it? What is its intensity on a scale of one to five? What color is it?

As you develop this heightened awareness, breathing deeply from center, you will notice that your fear shifts and the tension in your body dissipates. You are moving away from the future and past, and into the present, where fear disappears.

When you need to take action, after being in fear, do so in small increments, so you can remain in the present moment. For example, if I'm working with a skier paralyzed with fear on a mogul run, I take the time to get him centered, and then ask him to ski one big easy turn and stop. He can then build from that one-turn-at-a-time sequence into two turns and then three, as he becomes comfortable. Before he knows it, he has skied the entire mogul run that previously had him frozen in fear.

It's important to know that as you get centered and present, your fear will shift into useful rather than abusive energy. Fear is a powerful opportunity to learn about yourself and become fully aware.

Hero

Center is not a narrow tightrope through life requiring stern effort.
Center is a spacious field of consciousness
Where the flowering of feelings is honored
As one flows compassionately along the path of purpose.

Heroes. They provide us with pictures and possibilities. In short, they inspire us and keep our sights high. And if our heroes are real enough, and our actions are aligned enough, our dreams can become reality. It's like a cosmic internet powered by intention and consciousness. No batteries required.

Heroes. I have had many. In my early youth I revered Sir Lancelot. Old dented trash can lids, sharp sticks, and a small scar on my left cheek spark instant flashbacks of my three-year reign as the Silver Knight. I worshiped the 1950s Washington Senators. Ask me to name the player at any position and I will. With three pieces of bubble gum in my eight-year-old cheeks, the radio turned up loud, and my Louisville Slugger held high above my shoulder, I became each player, pitch by pitch. If the Senators lost (and they often did), the bat would slam to the carpet, and off to the showers I would go. The showers of my tears. I cried a lot in those days. Just check the Senator's record.

Our heroes change as we do. We become less interested in

simple physical prowess and bravery and are more drawn to heroes who embody commitment, passion, and service. As I grew out of childhood, my heroes were harder to come by. At least the live ones. Were they no longer making heroes like they used to, or did I have higher standards? How wonderful it would have been to have listened to Socrates challenge his countrymen, to have witnessed Michelangelo on the scaffolding, studied under Einstein, served under Jefferson or Gandhi. They ignite dreams of our highest selves and inspire us to take action on those visions.

Are there heroes today? Must we look only to the past for great teachers? Is greatness only bestowed on a person after his death, when his contribution has passed the test of time and memories of his basic human frailties have faded? Doesn't it take greater awareness to honor the giants of today because their significance is often disguised by the typical eccentricities of human nature, hiding their true value from all but the most perceptive? Could it be that a paint-mixer for Michelangelo went unaware of his proximity to greatness, too busy judging his boss's moodiness? Buddha must have belched on occasion or forgotten a disciple's name or misplaced his begging bowl. How many times have we missed a Buddha in our own midst because we perceived basic human flaws as a denial of greatness? The only heroes who are not vulnerable to human nature are made of stone, and stand motionless while pigeons strut on their shoulders.

As we grow from childhood to a more experienced and wrinkled existence, the qualities that we demand from our heroes change. Rather than looking for fast feet and a strong body, we look for a depth of compassion, wisdom, and inner peace.

If I had the opportunity to sit at the foot of any contemporary hero to learn the art and practice of compassion, there would be no question as to my choice. It would be the Dalai Lama. I had long hoped to meet the exiled Tibetan leader but had never

9

given the idea too much energy, appreciating the globe-trotting schedule and necessary insulation from the public that any world leader and Nobel laureate requires these days. Just another dream. But once again, I stand in awe of the power of dreams becoming reality.

While traveling in Southeast Asia with Eri, I had the great fortune to give a presentation to a conference of the World Presidents Organization in Bali. Halfway through the conference I had taken a day off to spend some time in the jungle of the less populated island of Lombok. When I got back, I noticed the blinking message light on the phone in my room. Fred Chaney, one of the main organizers of the event, was informing me that the Dalai Lama had recently confirmed his acceptance of a long-standing invitation and had arrived at the hotel. It had been agreed that His Holiness would co-lead a session on meditation the next morning with Mitsuo Aoki, a Japanese-American philosopher-priest in his eighties and (gulp!) me! Did I have the time to meet privately with the Dalai Lama at 5 P.M.? *What?* Let me hear that message again. A dream come true, a private meeting with the Dalai Lama! But *co-leading* a session? What an honor. What an opportunity. What a *crisis.* I checked my watch. It was 4:45 P.M. This is the kind of timing I love. No time to worry or to overprepare. Just get centered, breathe, and respond. No time to consider what to wear, what to say. No time to plan how to impress His Holiness on the one hand, and in so doing, miss the entire moment on the other. I dashed out in my flowered shirt (the bargain warehouse variety from Hawaii), shorts, flip-flops, and wraparound sunglasses.

There were two monks in orange robes standing outside the Dalai Lama's door when I arrived. The gentleness and joy in their faces said what translations could not. They were happy to see me. Maybe they just liked my shirt.

We bowed, shook hands, and one of them said, "His Holiness will be with you in a moment."

A little time to spare and the first pang of anxiety hit me. What was the protocol? Shoes or no shoes? Take those stupid sunglasses off! Should I have brought a gift? How should I address him? Just as I was about to inquire, the door opened. The monk in the doorway bowed and stood to the side as a beaming face behind him engulfed me with love and compassion.

"Welcome," His Holiness said, holding out his hands for mine, as if he were my long lost grandfather. Of course, he kind of was.

He took my hand in both of his and bowed, looking at me with kindness that melted every residue of nervousness inside me. He led me by the hand into the room and into a chair. Placing his chair within a foot of mine, he sat down, leaned forward with his forearms informally collapsed on his knees, his smiling face alert and excited, as if he were visiting with a beloved relative, keen to hear every word of his adventures. I felt affirmed and acknowledged, not through words, but because he was fully present with me—not with his thoughts, his plans, or his opinions—but with me, the guy from Colorado with the loud shirt. And to be honest, from that moment on I can't remember a thing we talked about. Only that it was a profound time of peace and connection.

After a time, Fred Chaney and Mitsuo Aoki appeared in the room to discuss the next morning's session. We all looked to the Dalai Lama, but his happy expression said it all. Whatever we decided was fine with him.

Being quicker of thought than I, Mitsuo took the reins and suggested that he could make some opening remarks and then introduce the Dalai Lama. After the Dalai Lama had spoken, His Holiness would turn it over to me to do whatever Colorado ski bums like me would do in such a situation. Everyone seemed to approve of the concept except me. I took a deep breath and spoke.

"Excuse me, Your Holiness, but as much as I am honored by this opportunity, I have considerations. You see, I've been involved in the practice of meditation for only twenty years. I am a novice (sniff). You've been involved in the practice your entire lifetime, and, thousands of lifetimes prior to this one. I am deeply honored to be in your presence and that is enough. Anything I say may be unworthy. I do not need to do anything. And besides (insert whining music here), I think . . ."

It took only one penetrating look, a fatherly smile, and the wave of an arm for His Holiness to quiet my ramblings, dispel my fears, and confirm the original plan. I was in awe of the faith he had in the outcome without even knowing what Mitsuo or I was going to say or do. I had images of puncturing the spiritual balloon of Tibetan Buddhism for years to come. I saw myself gabbing on about how little white guys meditate, while long-deceased Tibetan monks turned over in their graves out of fear that somebody might think that they approved of this insanity. But my fears dissolved instantaneously as the Dalai Lama continued to beam at me with confidence and trust.

It was only that evening as I was going to bed that the worries began anew. But with each fret, I would recall the Dalai Lama's face—relaxed, compassionate, and full of joy. And I had to relax and let go. What else could I do?

In the morning I met Mitsuo a half hour early to go over the setup of the room. On the stage was a large circular dais for the Dalai Lama, with a simple chair on either side for Mitsuo and myself. Mitsuo had felt that this would be the best arrangement, and I concurred, as it allowed the center of attention to be on the Dalai Lama. When the audience was filled to capacity, a spokesperson informed the audience of the proper protocol. The arrival of His Holiness would be announced just prior to his entering the room. Everyone was to stand quietly until he had entered and sat. I noticed two men quickly climbing on the stage to replace the dais with a chair.

"What's the problem?" I overheard one of the organizers nervously ask one of the men.

"Oh, His Holiness has asked that he not be put above the two others, as he never wants to be treated in a superior manner if at all possible."

"Of course," I thought, seeing that grandfatherly image of him again in my mind.

"His Holiness, the Dalai Lama," came the announcement.

Everyone stood up quickly with hushed excitement. Mitsuo and I stood by the door, ready to follow him up on stage after he was seated. But, as soon as he entered, he went right to us with that relaxed, almost sheepish grin, and those ever-kind eyes. Taking each of us by the hand, he led us onto the stage with him. There we were—the revered Tibetan monk, an elderly Japanese priest, and a little guy from Colorado—traipsing across the stage hand in hand. The Dalai Lama had made sure that, despite our differences, we were on the same boat.

Mitsuo, a warm and energetic man who works extensively with the terminally ill, gave some eloquent comments about the auspicious nature of the occasion. He then began to introduce His Holiness. All eyes shifted to the Dalai Lama, who was leaning forward and looking at the audience as if he had just found a precious flower and didn't want to miss any of its beauty.

As Mitsuo began to describe the grace and dignity of His Holiness, the Dalai Lama reached into his robe and took out a handkerchief. He turned to the side discreetly to blow his nose, unaware that his microphone was directly beneath his nose. The magnified snorting that followed resounded through the room like a cow in labor. The crowd, not having been informed of any nose-blowing protocol, sat in polite but embarrassed silence. The introduction continued, and amazingly so did the Dalai Lama's nose-clearing. And then suddenly, after one more foghorn blast, His Holiness realized that the thunder he was hearing was his own. He slowly, with his head still tilted, turned to the audience very sheepishly and broke into a face-consuming grin. He looked like a little kid caught in a peekaboo game.

71

9

The audience laughed uproariously, releasing all of its pent-up anxiety. Without a word spoken, His Holiness had created instant rapport. The day before, he had demonstrated trust and compassion for me. Now he was demonstrating the love he had for himself.

His Holiness spoke of the importance of meditation, and the daily practices of kindness and gratefulness, a lesson he had already taught me several times over. As I watched him speak so simply and profoundly, I recognized a living example of a truly centered man who walks his talk. A man who has not had it easy—whose people have been slaughtered by the hundreds of thousands, whose six thousand monasteries have been brutally destroyed, and who has been in exile for four decades. Literally, here was a man without a country. And yet he possessed no apparent hatred, no animosity toward the Chinese. He knew intuitively that no value can be added by such a reaction and it would be himself who suffered most if he were to justify anger and resentment in the place of kindness.

Eventually, it was my time to speak. I had been so immersed in the quality of His Holiness's being that the ego-demons of fear were cleansed. It was easy to be centered in his presence. I stood up and shared two stories that I felt were embodied by the Dalai Lama.

The first concerned an arrogant sixteenth-century samurai. In the strict class system of ancient Japan, any show of disrespect to a samurai was met, at the minimum, with a scolding or, at worst, immediate beheading. This particular samurai had been wandering through the village, growing increasingly irritated as he heard endless glowing acknowledgments of a revered monk named Takuan.

Finally, the jealous samurai shouted, "Where is the monk? We'll just see what he has to teach me!"

The villagers said that he lived in the forest high on a mountain above the village. The samurai proceeded to climb to the mountain. When he reached the top, he searched the forest until he finally came upon a monk who was sitting quietly under a tree.

"So, you're the monk they talk about. Well, monk, tell *me* the difference between heaven and hell."

The little monk looked up at him and said with a smile, "Get out of here. You disgust me. You're despicable. You have no right to even call yourself a samurai."

Enraged at the monk's evident display of disrespect, the samurai drew his sword and was about to cut the monk's head off when the monk calmly raised his hand and said, "That is hell."

Now at this the samurai dropped his sword. In such awe that this little monk had the courage and the willingness to end his life in order to teach, he dropped to his knees.

As the samurai bowed in gratitude, the monk smiled once more, raised his hand, and said softly, "And that is heaven."

I looked at the Dalai Lama, who had been chuckling and nodding his head with appreciation for the story.

"I'd like to share one more story that was said to have taken place in your homeland of Tibet."

The story took place during Alexander the Great's reign over the Asian Empire. The lieutenants of Alexander's army had scoured the countryside, requiring all the religious factions to pledge their allegiance to the empire. Upon their return the lieutenants reported to their general that everyone had pledged allegiance except for one little monk who lived high in a mountain village. Enraged, the general donned his armor and rode his horse at top speed to the village, where he found the little monk meditating under a tree.

He jumped off his horse, clambered over to the monk, and looked down on him, "Do you realize *who I am*? Do you know that I could draw my sword and cut off your head without blinking my eye!"

The little monk looked up at the ferocious, pompous general with compassion. "And do you know who I am? Do you know that I could have you draw your sword and cut off my head without blinking *my* eye?"

When I finally hit my little bell to signal the time for silent meditation, the image of the centered man sitting next to me appeared in my mind. Here also was such a man, unblinking in the face of death, not staring down his enemy with defiance but gently disarming him with the strength of his compassion. Even in my most outrageous dreams I can't come up with heroes like this.

I slept and dreamt that life was joy
I awoke and saw that life was service
I acted and behold!
Service was joy.

—*RABINDRANATH TAGORE*

EXPLORE YOUR TRUE SELF

The authenticity of a Dalai Lama reflects a deep knowing of center. Being centered allows you to tell the truth in a simple way. From a centered state, there is no need to exaggerate who you are and what you are doing in order to get approval. You recognize very clearly that who you are is enough, you don't have to add more than the universe has already given you.

There is an old Zen phrase: "If you understand, things are just the way they are. If you do not understand, things are just the way they are." So to be centered is to experience things the way they are and to not fear perceptions. Center builds confidence in your connection to all of life, and an acceptance of what life brings.

Living from center on a daily basis is certainly enhanced by the discipline of meditation. Becoming quiet in a busy world is something we would all love to do. One of the difficulties that many people have in considering meditation is that they think it is one more thing that they have to do in their life, another entry on that great list of things to do, such as working out, eating right, being on time, doing your job well. But meditation practice is not an effort, it is non-doing. It is a time to spend each and every day in that place inside yourself in which there is deep security and peace. So meditation is not some stoic physical position or arduous mental exercise. It is really a letting go. It is a joyous gift.

Taking the time to meditate daily will actually save you time in the end because of the increased clarity you gain. But, since the normative system doesn't hit a gong at 8 A.M. or 5 P.M. for the world to settle down and return to its higher self, you have to establish the practice. This is where the discipline takes place.

All cultures are steeped in an esoteric practice of one form or another to help people get in touch with that higher aspect of themselves. In the Judeo-Christian tradition, it is contemplative prayer—quietly residing in the presence of God rather than throwing out a list of demands or requests as if writing to Santa Claus. In the Far Eastern traditions the vehicles of meditation often have to do with the autonomic aspects of the nervous system, such as breathing or the heartbeat. In India, mantras from Sanskrit are used as a vehicle to take us inside (such as in Transcendental Meditation, a classical technique taught throughout the world). In the Zen Buddhist tradition, it is sitting with awareness of thoughts without clinging to them. In all of these disciplines the practice is not to force yourself into a state of peace, it is simply to acknowledge the mind's thinking nature and to relax into center so that you can settle down into deeper levels of thought, to the source of thought where the vibrational level is most powerful. It is achieving a place of deep connection and tranquillity, where you are accessing a field of intelligence that is far greater than that derived from ego and intellect.

When exploring an art you know very little about, whether it be meditation, playing the piano, or auto mechanics, trust your own center regarding choosing a teacher or support group. No matter what the art, good teachers should be compassionate, caring, and enthusiastic about what they do. They have fun and are continually exploring and learning themselves. They walk their talk (remember they don't have to be perfect) and most of all, they encourage you to think for yourself. This is very important in learning meditation because the practice is a daily inquiry into *your* true nature, not theirs.

Often people give up a valuable meditation practice because they don't understand the role of thoughts in the process. They think they shouldn't have thoughts during meditation, or that only certain thoughts are appropriate. The mind works through the medium of thoughts. Trying to deny them in meditation is like telling a person, "Close your eyes and don't think of mosquitoes." Often in meditation people try to control and fit their meditation into a certain picture or expectation of what meditation should be. Meditation is a letting-go process, an exploration into the source, the nature of mind. You can't explore the unknown by hanging on to what you think you know already.

The mechanics of meditation is similar to sleeping. When sleeping, you first get light rest, then deep rest. It's at the level of deepest rest that stress is released most powerfully. Your body begins to shift, align, and heal. This takes physical activity. Since the mind and body are connected, the mind also becomes activated, and this flow of thoughts we call dreams. These thoughts, or dreams, are simply the by-product of the release of stress. As they pass, we return to deep sleep and the cycle repeats itself.

Similarly, in the meditation cycle, thoughts are part of the stress-release process. They shouldn't be analyzed or used to evaluate whether the process is good, bad, or neutral. Thoughts are healthy and natural, and there is no need to judge yourself with statements such as, "I wish I could stop thinking long enough to meditate."

When thoughts surface during your meditation, don't get caught up in them. Know that they are all part of the practice, and a good part. Simply return to your meditation vehicle, whether it is the breath, a mantra, or a simple thought about God. It will nurture you and take you deeper into your meditation. Just keep letting go and letting God. Isn't this the essence of true prayer?

The only way to evaluate a meditation practice is on the quality of your life after about six months of regular practice of twenty to thirty minutes, once or twice a day. Are you more joyful, aware, compassionate, and centered than before? Drop by drop in an effortless manner, you are discovering your true self.

If you knew each day that you could relax in Mother's arms and be nurtured and rocked to health and vitality, wouldn't you do it? This is the gift of letting go.

Explore the various meditative techniques and support groups in your area. Meditation is not a religion, it is a way to bring you into greater awareness of your spiritual essence, and will deepen your personal religious affiliation. Explore and experiment, but by all means give yourself the daily gift of going inside to let go and let God.

The B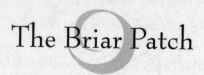iar Patch

Center is not a place.
It's a state of being
Where decisions are known,
not made.

Many years ago I took my first two aikido sensei (sensei means "teacher," and to refer to someone in this manner shows respect and honor), Rob Kobayashi Sensei and Koichi Tohei Sensei, to a high mountain lake above my home in the Colorado Rockies. Koichi Tohei was from Tokyo and at the time was chief instructor under Morehei Ueyshiba, the founder of aikido. In the calm peaceful surroundings Tohei Sensei reflected on one of his most important learnings about center.

"Centering saved my life in World War II," he told us. "I didn't want to be there fighting."

Tohei spoke of his responsibility for leading his men deep into mainland China. Potential ambushes loomed at every turn. In addition, Tohei also faced a moral dilemma. He believed in the tenets of aikido, to create peace and protection for all living things. Killing was reprehensible to him. Tohei's route through China was neither specific nor predetermined. How could he carry out his mission of penetrating the enemy's borders and yet still preserve life?

Tohei was very young-looking for an officer. To lead his men, he knew he would have to gain their respect. In the first firefight that they encountered, they found themselves taking shelter in a trench. The men would peek their heads up, shoot quickly and randomly before ducking down again. Tohei knew that someone needed a better perspective on the battle and that it had to be him. He harnessed his past aikido training, got centered, and stood up in the trench to better follow the battle. And he continued to "feel" or sense from his center. When a certain clear rush of off-centeredness occurred, he would duck back down. Often this uncentered feeling was followed immediately by enemy fire. His center had somehow been able to anticipate the attack prior to the actual shooting. His men began to draw courage from him and to deeply respect this man's willingness to face danger.

Later, on the march again, Tohei used the same centering powers to choose directions. When that uncentered state would occur, he would breathe deeply and try to regain center. When it did not come back, he would choose another direction, and if he regained that centered feeling, he would continue on the new path.

Occasionally, Tohei's troop would capture enemy soldiers. Tohei would take away their weapons and, as a show of his desire for peace, release the prisoners at nightfall. Many times thereafter, Tohei and his men would come across the enemy troops in the distance. Recognizing this peaceful man, the enemy would simply wave from across the field and allow Tohei and his men to pass. If this weren't remarkable enough, Tohei returned from China having lost none of his men and, according to his memory, having harmed no one.

Like Tohei Sensei, my son and I were caught in a war during

our Southeast Asian adventure; unlike Tohei Sensei, we didn't even know it.

It all began in Bali, ironically one of the most peaceful places on earth. Some environments present a real challenge to be centered. Bali makes it easy. The Balinese people have a delicate balance of warmth and royalty that I'd never encountered before. Their ancestral roots embrace many cultures and their unique blend of Buddhism, Hinduism, and island animism results in a hospitality that leaves you feeling honored. (And well fed!) Missing is the sense of animosity so often felt in other countries where there is a great disparity between the people and the obvious material riches of the tourists.

The Balinese seem to recognize the sacredness of life as an essential ingredient for happiness, and even while at work in the rice paddies or building roads, their movements embody a distinct grace. Women roadworkers carry eighty pounds of rock on their heads with the dignity of a princess going to her coronation. There is a conscious integration of work, worship, and celebration. Everything from rainy season to death is honored through art, dance, and ritual. I realized that I was not in a land where many artists live, but in a land where everyone is an artist.

It was hot and exotic in Bali. The Indian Ocean was a bath that you could lie in all day. Eri and I had traveled through the exquisitely lush countryside, captivated by the Balinese people and their clothing, temples, crafts, and customs. One evening we laid on a fine sand beach getting massaged by a couple of strong-handed, gentle-souled Balinese women.

I was preoccupied with an invitation I had received a few days earlier. A good friend from the Philippines, Robbie Delgado, had asked me to do a workshop for his organization in Manila. He suggested that it would be an opportunity for Eri to visit another beautiful country. Robbie was a good friend and I didn't want to let him down. After all, we were already in Southeast Asia and the opportunity to visit the Philippines might not come up again. I could use the work to help pay for our trip. On the other hand, it would be hard to leave Bali, so soothing to the body and soul. Ah, decisions, decisions! We left the next day.

As we landed in Manila, I felt increasingly uneasy. The humid, smog-covered city, with crowded streets full of thousands of impoverished people, was oppressive. Entire families lived in makeshift homes on the medians of major roads, surviving on whatever they could obtain from begging and hustling. In juxta-position were supermodern buildings and limousines, big dollars waving in the face of poverty, all the conditions needed to provoke hostility and revolution.

As we pushed our way through some beggars, the uneasy feeling persisted. When Tohei Sensei had an uneasy feeling, he used his center to choose a correct path, rather than adhering solely to the rational mind or to the fickle nature of emotions. We sat down on a bench and breathed deeply. And in the calm quiet that followed, I knew that we had to leave Manila. The workshop wasn't for several days and we could return then. Robbie, being the ever-gracious host, suggested the town of Baguio, approximately two hundred miles to the north, in the high, rugged, and spectacularly lush mountains.

Within hours we were at the airport for the one-hour plane ride to Baguio. The mountains and scenery were indeed spectacular and, as fortune would have it (or is it center?), we found ourselves at the Baguio Country Club, where we entered golf heaven, our room overlooking the first tee. During our first round we teamed up with a Filipino man named Victor. He said that the town would be crowded in a couple of days as the country club was hosting the Fil-Am Open, one of the biggest amateur golf tournaments in Asia. Teams would be coming from as far away as Japan, Australia, Taiwan, and Guam. Both courses would be closed for three days, beginning Friday. No problem for us, I thought, as we were leaving on Thursday for Manila and my upcoming workshop.

On Thursday morning we took a cab to the airport terminal. It had been a great few days. I was centered and ready for the heat and hustle of Manila. But, as we drove into the Baguio airport, I noticed how strangely desolate it looked. No one was around, no cars, no people, no planes on the runway. A ghost town.

"I guess we're the only ones on the flight," I said to Eri as we unloaded our bags and proceeded to the terminal door.

Suddenly, a young solider with an assault rifle approached us. There was no one else in the terminal.

"Sorry, sir, but the airport is closed. There is a war going on and the rebels have seized the airport in Manila," he said matter of factly.

Ah, a war. Is that all? Apparently he didn't understand that I had a workshop to give.

There was a sense of urgency on his face. I looked at his assault rifle. I decided not to file a complaint.

Whose side is he on? I thought, but felt it prudent to hold my question. Whose side am *I* on?

"When did this happen?" I asked, marveling at how isolated one can be from significant events. If the world as we know it had ended, how long would it take to get the message up here in the Philippine mountains? I mean, could we get in another eighteen holes before we felt it?

"Only two hours ago. There is fighting in Manila now," he said, and walked away.

Eri and I stood side by side in front of the empty terminal, stunned.

"Can you imagine if our plane had left an hour earlier? We would have been on the runway in Manila when the airport takeover happened. Is this timing coincidence, or are we blessed?"

We were definitely grateful. Had my center known a few days before when we made the auspicious decision to leave Manila? Was this what Tohei Sensei had been talking about?

Now what? Eri and I felt suddenly alone. We could possibly rent a car and negotiate the mountainous four-hour drive ourselves. We decided to go back to the hotel and check with Robbie in Manila on the status of things. During the cab ride back the first option was immediately canceled.

"The one and only road out of Baguio had been cut off by the military and there are soldiers and checkpoints everywhere," said the driver.

"Who are these rebel forces involved in the war?" I inquired.

"People in the military," was the reply.

Of course, I thought, it's almost always the military against the military because they are the ones with the weapons and the inside info.

"But how can you tell the difference between the government forces and the rebel forces?" I asked.

"You can't," laughed the cabdriver.

And now I was more confused than ever. One thing was for certain. If the rebels had taken over the Manila airport and therefore the Filipino air force that was also stationed there, this was not a small inefficient operation. Airpower is a huge trump card in the war game.

Arriving back at the hotel, we found a message from Robbie saying that he would do everything to get us out of the country but for now we had no other choice but to stay put. He advised us not to wander too much in town, and that he had made arrangements for us to stay at the golf club until it was safe to leave. Eri and I returned to our rooms. As we stood on our porch overlooking the first hole, we began to sense the sheer lunacy of our predicament. Here we were, two fanatic golfers, held captive in a foreign country during a coup d'état, where else but at a country club with full golf privileges and all

9

expenses paid. The management announced that they did not recommend that Americans (we were the only ones) leave the premises but that we could play all the golf we wanted. Uncle Remus and Br'er Rabbit were for real. We convulsed with laughter at the briar patch we'd been thrown into.

"War is hell," I said to Eri a few minutes later as we were teeing it up. We could be the only POWs ever released with suntanned grins and scratch handicaps.

Each evening we emerged from the golf trenches, battle-weary from hooks and shanks, to watch CNN's version of the coup and compare it with Robbie's phone messages, coming from the middle of the action in Manila. CNN kept claiming that President Corazon Aquino had things in control, but Robbie kept reporting just the opposite. We discovered that the building that we had originally planned to use for the workshop in Manila had become the headquarters of the rebellion and that most of the shooting was in and around that building. Our cup of gratefulness for being in Baguio was overflowing. Trusting in my center had paid off. It had taken us from a dangerous rifle range in Manila to a pleasurable driving range in Baguio.

It *was* disconcerting to find young kids with rifles guarding the doors of the restaurant when we went to eat. There are few aikido techniques for automatic weapons. First monkeys, then elephants, now automatic weapons. I have a lot to learn.

And in truth, we learned rather quickly that it is not the automatic weapon that we need to be aware of. Instead, we need to be aware of the man holding it. Our smiles, simple hellos, and common courtesies were far better than a flak jacket.

Each day things became more precarious (which probably only added to the degree of slice that was developing in my golf swing). President Aquino was fervently asking for the United States to intervene militarily and quash the uprising. President Bush's upcoming decision whether to invade was a critical one with regard to our security. Would these two blond-haired Yankees enjoy such a warm reception if our American brothers started bombing their Filipino brothers?

You must remember that military coups happen in the Philippines with such frequency that they are sort of like elections in the United States. The electorate just happens to use guns instead of ballots. Getting out the vote had an entirely different meaning there. But that is precisely why it is usually not appropriate for a foreigner to intervene. It became obvious that regardless of which side the Filipinos were on, they would come together quickly against the United States if we got involved militarily. Half-jokingly, Eri and I began to practice Swedish accents, knowing that our Colorado twangs would not cut it in the aftermath of a decision by President Bush to bomb the rebels.

Within a few days our prayers must have been heard because President Bush turned down Aquino's request for bombing runs. Instead, he provided a military assurance that Philippine airspace was off-limits to the rebels, eliminating their ability to use the Philippine air force to their distinct advantage. Relief! We could breathe again. I could see my slice straightening already.

Meanwhile, what had happened to the largest amateur international golf tournament in Asia with its hundreds of entries? A large percentage of the entrants had shown up for practice prior to the coup. And now the roads were closed. I quickly learned that the commitment of modern soldiers pales in comparison to the intensity of the committed golfer. Clearly, if there were more golfers, there would be fewer wars. Because if the choice is between a rifle and a five-iron, you want to be selling golf balls, not bullets. The question here was not whether or not they would have the tournament in the midst of the war. It was how could we keep the young kids with assault rifles off the greens. Or at least get them to repair their divots.

During that first day in Baguio our Filipino golfing partner, Victor, had been impressed by the smooth, flowing swing of the small young, blond American kid named Eri, not to mention the 75 that he shot. I'm sure my banana slices left him more dubious. Nevertheless, he invited us to join his all-Filipino team from the Wak Wak Country Club in Manila. They needed one more player and an alternate. There was no doubt about who would be the alternate. We gleefully accepted with the reservation that if the road opened and we had an opportunity to leave the country, we would have to go. Victor was delighted and there we were—bona fide members of the Wak Wak Filipino golf team in a small mountain village in the middle of a war. We'd be walking around the fairways with five-irons while young soldiers were walking along the adjacent streets with assault rifles. But the sight of nervous kids in army green wasn't nearly as intimidating as the fierce stares of my competitors as I lined up a five-foot putt.

And we still weren't sure whose side anybody was on. You see, in most wars you know who the enemy is. But in coups in the Philippines, everyone wears the same uniform with the exception that the rebels wear armbands. The intriguing thing was, they would put the armbands on only when they thought it best. You can see the difficulty of regulating such a war. These coups can drag on for weeks, and everyone knew it would happen again whenever people got sufficiently frustrated with the economy, the inability to live a productive life, and the tremendous disparity between haves and have-nots. But, since neither side had called me in to help resolve the conflict, I was restricted to remain in golf heaven. I accepted my fate. And three days later our team was winning the whole damn tournament.

On the last day of the tournament, the long-awaited phone call came. We were to meet a car and driver outside the hotel who would drive us to Manila immediately. There would be military checkpoints along the way, but we should have no trouble. This was the most appropriate time to leave, and things could get considerably worse later. So the time was now.

Shoot! The call finally comes for our freedom and safety and we don't want it. The Fortieth Annual Men's Fil-Am International Golf Tournament is at stake and we are in first place! Let's get our priorities straight here. Continue the roadblock for just one more day so we would have no conflicting thoughts to screw up our backswing. But, alas, after conferring with our Filipino teammates, and returning to center in quiet meditation, the answer became clear. We should leave during the lull.

So off we went, our new-found friends waving their golf hats at us, thanking us (Eri) for our (his) strong contribution.

Within twenty-four hours we had hugged our hero and savior Robbie Delgado good-bye at the Manila airport and were rising once more above the deep blue Pacific, the war-torn Philippine islands in the distance. Par/birdie blessings to our Team Filipino, and may they be wearing the right colored armband when the rifle smoke clears. We had followed our centers. Instead of being hostages in a firefight in Manila, we had been forced to play golf for eight days in the mountains.

It is all starting to hang together. It took ghetto kids and snowstorms, the monks and monkeys, the jungle treks and coup attempts to get a handle on a few simple words. Without real-life experiences, they are just nice words on a philosophical bookshelf. With them the words are a source of strength for a lifetime. *Listen to Your Center. Let Go and Let God. But! Tie Your Camel!*

A half year later I was halfway around the world from the Philippines doing a keynote presentation at the Orlando Convention Center for the National Conference of the American Society for Training and Development. At the end of my presentation a backstage assistant informed me that there was a man who would like to see me. I couldn't believe my eyes. There stood Victor, with a beaming smile and a big paper bag in his hands. I rushed over to embrace him and watched as he brought from the bag a gigantic two-foot trophy, in two parts, one in each hand.

"I'm sorry it broke," he yelled, "but we took third place!"

But anywhere is the center of the world.

—*Black Elk*

BE "PRESENT IN THE MOMENT"

The revered Buddhist monk Thich Nhat Hanh once taught a seminar during which, every few minutes, helicopters from a nearby construction project flew overhead. Instead of treating this as a disruption, he made it an opportunity to be centered, to be mindful. At the sound of a helicopter, dialogue would halt, and everyone would center. He taught the participants to frame the noise as an asset, not a liability.

You don't need a beautiful monastic setting to appreciate center. In fact, the power of center may be more apparent in chaos. Trapped in a coup d'état in the Philippines, or commuting on a subway in New York can be excellent places to get centered. It's not about time or location, it is about intention.

The busier and more frantic your life, the more rigorous you could be about remembering to center. The busy moments and crazy times can be a signal to say "Aha, time to center." During rush hour, in the boardroom, or when your kindergartner is throwing a tantrum are exactly when you have an opportunity to recapture center and act with renewed calm and focus.

On the sweatshirts and T-shirts of my company and on the logo of all our mailings, we have a little strawberry. That strawberry is a symbol, a reminder to center. The strawberry actually comes from an old samurai story. It is about a samurai who is chased by a bear. He literally runs off a cliff. As he's falling, he grabs a branch.

He looks up and sees the bear leaning over the cliff, clawing at his head, missing only by inches. As he looks down to the ground below, only about fifteen feet, he sees a lion leaping up, missing his feet only by inches. As he looks at the branch he is clutching, he sees two groundhogs gnawing away at it. He watches as his lifeline disappears, bite by bite.

As he centers and takes a deep breath, he notices, next to his branch, a clump of wild strawberries. In the midst of the clump is a great, red, juicy strawberry. With his one free hand, he reaches over, picks the strawberry, puts it in his mouth, chews slowly and says, "Ah—delicious."

Now when I tell that story to most western audiences, they find it confusing. They want to know what happened next. The point is that when you are able to get centered, you are truly in the moment, able to enjoy that strawberry, and it is in that moment of full awareness that you will do what is most appropriate in dealing with the lions and the bears and the groundhogs. In a very busy, frenetic life, when you remember to center and enjoy the strawberry, you can watch the stress, struggle, and emptiness drop away.

Part II

Uh-oh!

The water before, and the water after,

Now and forever flowing, follow each other.

If you wish to know the road up the mountain,

You must ask the man who goes back and forth on it.

The wild geese do not intend to cast their reflection;

The water has no mind to receive their image.

Like a sword that cuts, but cannot cut itself;

Like an eye that sees, but cannot see itself.

Draw water, and you think the mountains are moving;

Raise the sail, and you think the cliffs are on the run.

Entering the forest he moves not the grass;

Entering the water he makes not a ripple.

—*Zenrin*

Back in the USA

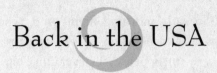

Only in the center of the storm is it calm.
But it takes courage to go there.

In the jungle of Southeast Asia, the monk and monkeys made centered life look easy. But back in the rat race of our ultramodern jungles, it's a different texture of mud. Instead of stumbling about in swampy elephant holes, one flounders in the frenetic whirlpool of commerce and commercials. Instead of dodging slithering creatures, one must deal with crazed two-legged mammals.

We had been flying for twenty-some hours. Eri and I staggered out of customs with a few functioning but raw brain cells left. This was not a good time to suggest to your teenager that he wash his baseball cap, or stand up straight. No, just keep a lid on what was left of sanity and check into your hotel.

Standing at the end of the check-in line, I noticed a potbellied businessman whom I had witnessed earlier on the plane knocking back several cocktails. He was trying to talk to the receptionist. Irritation was on him like poison ivy, with much fidgeting, glancing frequently at his watch, and shaking of the head. He probably had an early morning flight. And, who knows, but maybe his bags never showed up, his wife had just left him, and his toenails were unclipped. Whatever, this big guy was not ready to party. The receptionist could sense the active volcano in front of her. Afraid to look him in the eye, she welcomed him coolly with a proper professional voice, "Good evening, sir." The right words but guarded, the way you might talk with a stranger on a New York subway. The guy looked more irritated than ever.

Customers hate it when no one is home. She was a human tape recorder on automatic. With an insincere smile she presented him with one of those infamous plastic key cards and told him his room number. Exhausted, the guest staggered to the elevator. My hunch says he got to his floor, stepped out, blindly made a wrong turn, and walked trancelike down an endless, slightly nauseating, multicolored hallway, designed by a sadist under the influence of hallucinogens.

On the second lap around, he probably saw what he remembered as his room number. "Finally," he must have muttered, sticking the dastardly plastic into the slot. But the little red light on the lock would have continued to blink. Cursing, maybe he would try flipping the card, but with no success. After several minutes of jiggling, jostling, and jerking the doorknob off its screws, he would glance at his watch: 1:15 A.M. He probably had a 7 A.M. flight. And his toenails still weren't clipped.

I was just getting my own amazing plastic gizmo from the receptionist when the raging bull emerged from the elevator and stormed to the front of the line. I quickly stepped aside, like any good spectator would do, knowing that I was about to receive more data for my ongoing study of center.

Conflict! It happens everyday in business and relationships, doesn't it? How did the hotel receptionist handle the raging bull? Well, let's first look at how she *might* have handled it.

We must consider that there might be a mixed bag of conflicting beliefs in the receptionist's head. For one, the hotel might have long emphasized the importance of customer service as the highest priority, which could be interpreted as "the customer is always right." But maybe the receptionist also had the belief that it's important not to be abused in life and she must stand up strong in the face of an attack.

The raging bull was foaming at the mouth and raving on about the despicable quality of service at the hotel. If uncentered, our matador receptionist might have had just enough assertiveness training to be dangerous. She would stop him in his tracks with her razor-sharp matador pic: "Sir, there is no need to be so upset. The key is simple to use. You take this side with the arrow pointing in, push it all the way in until you hear a discernible 'clunk,' and . . . blah, blah, blah."

This would make the guy salivate. He would now want to kill her, if only to end the lecture on Door Opening 101. A verbal battle would rage while time was wasted and toenails grew.

But maybe our beleaguered receptionist took a different approach. Maybe she would cower in the presence of the snarling bull. Of course, her chances of walking away with the seat of her pants unhorned would decrease drastically. Each weak little reply, regardless of the actual words, would sound like, "I'm sorry. I'm stupid. The whole hotel is stupid. Yell at us again because we deserve it." And, of course, the customer would keep chasing his retreating victim, like a Doberman on the attack.

Or maybe she tried to be centered, but misinterpreted centering. She, like many of us, might have mistaken it as a stoic death march through life, detached from all feelings and relationships. The man would shout and scream. And the receptionist would stare at him with a zombie expression, periodically monotoning, "Yes, sir. Go on, sir. I feel your pain, sir."

He would grab her by the neck and . . . (Just kidding. But wouldn't he like to?)

So, which approach did the receptionist choose in the face of this storm? Would she fight back, shrink, or feign detachment?

None of the above. Before she could even begin to react, a short, plump lady in her mid-fifties emerged from the office door located directly behind the receptionist. Her beaming, round face reminded me of the peaceful little monk in Southeast Asia. In a pleasant, enthusiastic voice, she jumped right into the middle of his harangue.

"You know, I just hate it when those little cards start acting up. And things like that always seem to happen just at the end of a tough day."

The man gawked at her in silence. His white-knuckled grip on the counter relaxed and his menacing grimace softened. She quickly grabbed another card from behind the counter and walked around to where he was standing. She lightly took him by the elbow and began leading him to the elevator.

"Let's get this taken care of right away."

And the man, as if in a trance, began to tag along beside her, like my Labrador retriever, Maggie, when you scratch her in just the right place.

People don't fight when there's no one to fight with. I used to try to throw a tantrum in front of my mom. But in the face of her understanding and love, my anger would dissipate.

"Sounds like it's been a tough day," she would say. "Wanna see what's baking in the oven?"

Suddenly, there was no one to fight, no payoff for my abusive behavior. And, the next thing you know, I'd be sitting at the kitchen table with a glass of cold milk and a plate of warm cookies.

All right, you might be saying, normal angry folks can be worked with. But what about the real crazies? Good question.

People can be different. I never knew *how* different until I was invited to work with John Denver as his bodyguard. In the mid-seventies John was one of the top entertainers in the world, doing two shows a night to packed houses of 18,000 people in the Madison Square Gardens of the world. I figured that it would be good basic aikido training to protect him from adoring fans, control a few drunks or disorderlies from time to time, and spend some private time helping John develop the skill of centering to create peace of mind in the crazy world of celebrities. What I did not count on were all the irrational folks out there who were trying to get to him for one reason or another. I'm speaking of people who inhabit other realms of reality, forcing me to rely not on normal negotiation skills but on creative thinking. I needed to jump into their world without questioning whose reality was right.

For instance, what do you do when you get a call from the sheriff's office stating they've got a guy camped out at the town courthouse with two mules?

"He's taken two months to walk his mules from Missouri to Aspen, and he's not about to leave until he sees John Denver," said the deputy. "Could you come over and talk some sense into this guy?"

I grabbed my jacket and pedaled my bicycle down Main Street to the courthouse. With my deep awareness, it was pretty easy to spot the guy. He was sitting on a bale of hay. He was the only guy there. And the only one with mules. A wiry man in his thirties with a full beard, dirty overalls and workshirt, lovingly stroking his mules.

"How ya doing?" I said nonchalantly as I cruised to a stop alongside him.

"Fine. How about you?" came the pleasant reply.

Whew! I was always relieved when the person was pleasant. An on-the-edge, violent tendency was usually communicated in the voice. But not always. It was sometimes disguised, but rarely well enough that you couldn't notice it in the eyes, the subtle twitches, the uncomfortable movement of the body (automatic weapons were also a clue). He passed the voice check. But, hey, when a guy walks all the way from Missouri with two mules, he is worthy of much closer scrutiny. As to his tendency toward the strange, there was no doubt. My fundamental interest was clear: Was he dangerous? And what would it take to defuse him if he were? And how could I best serve him? And what would happen if his demands weren't met?

I held out my hand, "My name's Tom. Mind if I sit and chat for a spell?" I was working on my midwestern farmer accent.

"No problem. Have a seat," he said graciously, motioning to another bale. I sat, and started chewing on a piece of hay. I always love doing that. Brings out the cowboy in me. We exchanged the normal pleasantries about weather. I asked about the personality of mules, and what he was doing in town. He was noncommittal on that one.

"Oh, just staying for a while. Came from Missouri."

"On those mules?"

"Yep, avoiding the interstates makes mule traveling a lot tougher."

I laughed. I liked this guy, even though I could see in his somber attitude he was on a quest. I looked into his intense eyes. He had that "I'm on a mission from God" look. And that always scared me. Pleasantries over, and rapport created, I decided to get to the point.

"I'm a friend of John Denver's. The sheriff's department told me that you are here to see him. I'm impressed to hear that you came from Missouri with two mules. Have you contacted John about this?"

"Nope, it wasn't necessary. I had to do it this way."

It was a sure sign that God was involved.

"Well, John's out of town now. But I'd gladly deliver a message for you." It was a stupid offer, but I thought I'd give it a shot.

"Nope. I've got to see him myself. I'll wait. I need to know the truth."

"What truth is that?" I prodded.

He examined me closely. I must have passed the test.

"Whether he's John the Baptist or not," he said, as if it should have been obvious to me. "It's important that he not hide it from the world anymore."

Whoa. Time to center. I knew I needed to pause to keep from arguing with him, which would have exacerbated the problem and created a loss of rapport. I needed to understand his viewpoint rather than judge it. I'd been here before. The double bind. To deny the accusation that John Denver was John the Baptist would have been useless. He would have concluded that I obviously wasn't a man of God, knowledgeable about such things. If I agreed with him about John, then he and his mules were certainly going to be in for a long stay. We would need a lot more hay. And a shovel.

I was certain that I had seen enough differences in perspective to know that I didn't know much, so who was I to argue such a point. Arguing only tends to produce greater conviction on the part of folks who walk a thousand miles with a couple of mules. No, he had his answer. John Denver and I either had to accept it or we were holding back the truth. I grabbed another long strand of hay and went through my mental files on similar situations.

Once I had been called on to try to talk sense into a woman who had holed up for three weeks in a one-room basement apartment in Aspen, knitting a quilt and refusing to leave her room until she could see John. She also had a different reality.

But as I sat on the floor for an afternoon talking to the quilt lady, I realized that different realities are as plentiful as cockroaches. The reality with the most advocates gets to be the standard for society. Who's to say that these fringe realities are *all* wrong? So I decided on an aiki approach with the quilt lady, to blend with rather than confront, to accept her premise that God had sent her to this basement to meet John, as strange as that thinking may seem. As I became willing to see her point of view, she began to see mine. I took a similar approach with the mule man.

The mule man wasn't really asking whether or not John Denver was John the Baptist. In his mind, he already knew. He just wanted John to declare it. The trouble with folks who have such strong convictions is that if John didn't admit to them, he would be performing some kind of deep wrong. And that, of course, was when I got concerned. Because if people feel that they are betrayed, especially on a mission from God, they may do radical things.

After a good deal of listening to his convictions, I saw an opening.

"Is John the Baptist a true man of God?" I asked.

"Of course," came the emphatic reply, "a very important one."

"Well, then, as a man of God, he must be constantly speaking to, and listening to, God for guidance. It must be incredible what John knows that I don't know, with all that direct connection to God."

"Yep."

I could see him nodding with approval.

"Then there must be a reason for John Denver to be withholding this kind of statement. God is guiding him to do this for a reason. It all must be for a good purpose. It's just that the purpose is yet to be known. God works in mysterious ways."

He was in deep thought.

"Yeah, God works in mysterious ways. But, it's up to John to tell us."

I looked for another straw to chew. There was still plenty in the bale.

"But why do you suppose God would keep John from saying anything? Maybe he's making a mistake."

"God doesn't make mistakes. He knows what He's doing," he snorted convincingly.

He had swallowed the bait. The mule man knew that John the Baptist would be following God's plan. And if he hadn't confessed his identity, then there must be a reason. After all, God doesn't make mistakes (except for turnips).

"Thank goodness God is in charge. I guess it makes John's life a lot more reassuring. God will let him know when the time is right."

I looked at him closely. The wheels were turning. There was no reaction of anger and betrayal, because *God* was in charge, which had been the mule man's reality to begin with.

I *am* glad he didn't ask, if that was the case, why the heck God sent him to Aspen via mules.

The same kind of reasoning had worked with the quilt lady, also on a mission from God. I never saw either one again. The apartment was vacated and the hay bales deserted after our talks. God does work in mysterious ways.

Of course, it wasn't always so clean and simple. One other case took a number of years to break through. It all started with a series of love letters to John. No big deal—it was happening by the bagful in those days—but if they got too insistent, bizarre, or voluminous (book-size), J.D.'s secretary would toss them in the "outward-bound" file and send them to me. Because of the urgency and demanding nature of one particular wheelbarrow load from a very devoted individual, I made the mistake of responding. And then she started writing to *me* instead of John. About John of course; I was her confidant. She was convinced that she and John were lovers, and that he had proposed marriage. I felt compelled to set the record straight. But with every clear, logical letter I wrote, describing John's wife and kids, I would receive more poetry and verse on her boundless love and

101

9

future marriage to John. I stopped responding, thinking that she would tire of such foolishness. But her letters kept coming. And then came the boxes of her belongings, including some very personal items! She was moving in!

At first I tried to return the belongings with terse letters of denial. But I was missing the point. She was living in a different reality, and I was fighting it rather than being centered enough to have the courage to explore it. To her it was simple—she and John were going to live together happily ever after, and she needed to move in.

I decided to accept her reality. And embellish it. So I wrote to her again. I thanked her for sending the belongings. I then indicated that a charitable organization that John supported did have a real need for certain items. They needed vehicles, washing machines, stereos, things like that. So if she really wanted to support John, would she please send her car, or maybe a television set, her toaster oven, perhaps her personal computer.

I have yet to receive any more letters or boxes. It has been over a decade, and times have changed. I might have to write again. We could use a new fax machine.

> *Yes: The young sparrows*
> *If you treat them tenderly*
> *Thank you with droppings.*

—*ISSA*

UNDERSTAND EMOTIONS

When an angry person confronts us, there is a tendency to contract. Instead of choosing a centered state, where we can see that the attacker is calling out for help, we contract into our own roller coaster of fear and pain. We often try to avoid this by fighting back or ignoring them completely. But when a door is slammed in an angry person's face, what is his typical reaction? To kick it in, of course. Or, if we get war-weary fighting them off and weakly acquiesce, we often find that the person continues their abuse upon us.

When we choose to be overly assertive, weakly compliant, or inappropriately detached, the angry person never feels heard. Temper tantrums, at any age, are often the result of feeling a lack of control, that no one is listening, nobody understands. When we react defensively, attack back, or show little caring, we are underscoring that message. And the tantrums only increase.

Centering allows you to receive fully what is being said and felt. To be centered is to feel emotions, to suspend your knee-jerk reaction to fight back or shrink. It allows you to cultivate a more expansive attitude. When you are centered, you feel a heightened sense of balance, relaxation, and calmness. You are able to recognize that we've all had bad days that push us over the edge into rage. That perspective can bring compassion and empathy to your interaction with an angry person. It will reflect in your body language, tonality, attitude, and ability to act. And when the angry person feels heard and understood, he will give up his tantrum, because he will know unconsciously that there is no war here, no unlistening doors to break down, or whining cries to egg him on. He can get quickly to his need without all the emotional bludgeoning. He has permission to feel his upset, without unleashing it on someone else.

But what if the angry person you are dealing with is yourself? When rage shows up, get centered, breathe deeply, and witness yourself—your physiology, your tone, your behavior. You will find you will still feel the emotion, but you will no longer be a victim of it, no longer operating out of it, nor raging at others. Any angry physiology and abusive behavior will dissipate and you will be able to discuss the source of your difficulties in a way that allows others to hear you.

Why? The centered state is a state of expansion, compassion,

103

connection; the uncentered state is a state of contraction, fear, separation, which shows up physically and emotionally as anger, apathy, depression. When you get centered, you are spacious enough to feel your emotions. They are no longer something you are, they are something you experience, like a weather pattern, which you realize will move on.

When centered in a conflict, you will be able to look inside and discover more of who you are and will want to use language that nurtures communication. Practice using "I" language, for example, when you're dealing with emotions. Instead of reacting in anger with "You're always late!" which usually leads to a defensive reaction from the other person, try "When I'm waiting I feel angry because I think our relationship isn't valued."

If your emotions are stated in a centered, authentic manner, you will not be misconstrued as blaming others. You will have minimized the possibility of a fight and maximized the opportunity for a dialogue.

It is important to know that emotions are energetic feedback about perceptions, not necessarily the truth about a particular situation. The feeling is indeed real, but it is based on a subjective judgment of a situation. Feeling upset when it snows may be true for someone in rush-hour traffic in a big city, but not for a skier in Colorado.

When we are constantly interpreting an emotion too quickly, and laying blame on ourselves or others, we can get caught in deeply rooted patterns of inappropriate behavior. For example, let's say a man grows up being taught that sadness is unmanly ("big boys don't cry"). Instead of centering and feeling sadness in a situation, he may react by lashing out at others, because he thinks he is failing as a man. Or say a woman is brought up to believe that she should never get angry, that it is unbecoming of a lady. When she feels anger as an adult, she might associate that with unworthiness, and adopt a weak, unwilling attitude or become passive aggressive.

With time, and daily centering practice, you will gain the ability to feel your real emotions rather than project adaptive behavior which serves no one. You will no longer feel compelled to deny your emotions or lash out at others or manipulate others because of them. Their energy can be released in beneficial and appropriate ways. Your upsets can be acknowledged and become platforms for learning. Your whole life becomes a conscious choice. And even in the midst of a tantrum, you can catch yourself, pause to center, and choose more conscious action. Whether you remember to catch yourself prior, during, or after the event, do it! It will always make a positive difference.

The Big Draw

Gowf is a mighty teacher never deviating from its sacred roots, always ready to lead us on. . . . And I say to ye all, good friends, that as ye grow in gowf, ye come to see the tings ye learn in every other place. . . . Ye'll come away from the links with a new hold on life, that is certain if ye play the game with all your heart.

—Shivas Irons, in Golf in the Kingdom by Michael Murphy

I'd first like to acknowledge myself, because I know what kind of courage it takes to admit that one is (gulp) addicted to golf. After all, isn't golf, as some wizened old pro once observed, a sadistic activity named by some dyslexic Scot who had meant to call it "flog"? I'm not sure how my addiction came about. I just know that golf and I are incongruous at best. I'm talking about a guy who grew up in the radical sixties, the age of protest, who swore off this neurotic pastime as a prime example of what was wrong with people in the world—cigar-chomping loonies wearing silly hats and even sillier checkered pants, driving here and there in little toy carts full of expensive garbage. Every minute or so, one would stumble from the cart with a metal stick ill-suited for its absurd purpose of putting a small round, dimpled ball into a hole somewhere in the middle of a converted cow pasture. As a man from the sixties generation, I had to wonder what those guys were smoking? They were playing on grass everyday and it was legal. I took great comfort in my disdain of the game.

Addicts usually blame someone or something else for their addiction. I've got to lay it all on my father (always a credible excuse) and his annual summer visit. It fascinated my two young sons to see their granddaddy don a pair of plaid shorts, calf-high dark socks, and a classy-looking fedora that shaded his twinkling eyes as he whisked off to the golf links. Or maybe it was the shoes—those multispiked white shoes that, in motion, sounded like a troupe of drunken tap dancers with bad attitudes. Or was it the array of metal weapons that he wheeled around? Whatever it was, it got the boys' attention.

So off we would go for our annual golf outing. Granddad with his bubbling enthusiasm would show the wide-eyed brothers the finer points of the swing. The boys would imitate him with clubs taller than they were. I would pace in the background, fighting off past images of failure in anticipation of the annual four hours of torture. Golf, after all, was stupid.

Now I've always thought of myself as a good athlete, having proven myself on athletic fields where *real* sports are played. Each summer I would venture out to the links to show the old geezer my superior power and sports finesse. But by the second or third hole I would find myself clear-cutting a major portion of a forest in a manic attempt to get that stupid little ball back onto the fairway where the old man had been all along. By the twelfth hole I would have lost four expensive balls and left two clubs on previous holes. Hours later I would limp to the eighteenth green, blistered, battered, and bewildered. Full-contact golf had been played. And as I would excavate my last chunk of ground swatting at the little round monster, I'd take inventory of my dad. His shirt would be dry, his clubs intact, and, knowing me as well as he did, he would be wise enough not to have too big a smile. He'd be standing on the green filling out the inevitable scorecard, that harmless little piece of paper that somehow had become more important than my IQ or any college diploma.

107

9

"I don't care about my score, Dad," I would lie as I stroked my putt directly at the hole, albeit ten feet short. I had clearly done the most work, but felt the worst. I was surrounded by absurdity, I thought, as I stroked my putt beautifully although this time ten feet too long.

Thank God, Dad would concede my next putt (more of a chip really), so I could finally put the clubs away until the next summer's outing.

I'm not sure how it happened, but years later I was hooked on this outrageous sport. I must have swallowed the bait one summer watching my old man drain a long snake of a putt for birdie. The connection between center training and golf hit me like a lightning bolt (maybe not the best metaphor in a golf story). It was crystal clear. Golf is an Art of Center.

Being a teacher of the martial arts had taught me the importance of calmness and being present in the moment. I hadn't fully realized it, but I had been on the lookout for a summer sport which, like snow skiing, could complement the art of aikido for me. I know in Japan that archery has been an excellent training in centering, but you can't simply drive into the average American city and flip through the yellow pages for the closest zen archery dojo. No, I needed a sport imbedded in mainstream America. But I never thought it would be golf!

Centering training helps us by stripping away the baggage of our lives—our tendency to cling to ego, to our belief systems, to our possessions—so we can become more aware of our true nature. Likewise, in golf it matters not what you believe or how many technological gimmicks you carry with you; the game has a way of leaving you naked, standing as a mirror before you, reflecting your deepest emotions and your most secret foibles. Watching a grown man going berserk brandishing a freshly broken putter makes you want to laugh and cry at the same time. It is a poignant image of the frailties of humanity. What an arduous path, through sand traps and rough, through trauma and travail, to pierce the essence of our true nature! What is the sound of one club snapping?

As Alan Watts says about a zen koan, after the frustration of contemplating it has stripped away your ego, there comes a flash of satori, a moment of enlightenment in which the disciple realizes that there was nothing in it after all! Nothing is left at this moment but to burst out into a good loud laugh.

Every golfer can relate to this buildup of frustration. But eventually there will come "the moment." Whack, and seemingly by divine intervention, a fading little sphere rockets through the blue sky and lightly touches down on a plush fairway hundreds of yards away. The golfer knows somehow in the effortlessness that he or she didn't hit it. Instead "It" hit it. "It" is the centered state—the state of muga—an absence of the feeling that "I'm doing it." One simply lets go and, voilà, it happens. The zen principle of mushin, or "no-mindedness," is what golfers call "the zone." And that one shot in the zone makes all the foundering worthwhile.

As you have already figured out, to describe center in words is to miss the mark. True center is the experience of being fully alive, not a description of that experience. You can't put wind in a box, or declare that a pail of ocean water is the ocean. Centering happens in the now, not in the future. Therefore, goals and expectations can't be of such importance that you miss the moment and the flow of the process. And when you think about it, rolling a little white ball into eighteen slightly bigger holes does seem rather pointless, don't you think?

For thousands of years Zen monks have contemplated koans such as "What is the sound of one hand clapping?" Somewhere in the process of trying to figure it out, the ego and intellect break down, and the Zen monk catches a fresh perspective of himself and the world. Aha! Could the endless struggle of the driver and putter provide a similar opportunity for enlightenment? (Driver and putter—yin and yang sticks? Am I getting out of hand, here?) But golf, like the Zen master's slap in the face, can be ruthlessly direct. It exposes one's ego and then destroys it. When we get lucky enough to birdie one hole, golf trashes our false sense of mastery with a triple bogey on the next.

As golf master Jack Nicklaus said, "You can never own golf. You only borrow it for a while."

It's helpful to be in nature when training in centering. The elements are marvelous teachers. Walking around a golf course can be like meandering through a botanical garden (or forest, or bog, or active lava field, if that's where the bounding white ball has led you). And on many courses near my home, deer, fox, gophers, and geese share the fairways with golfers. The U.S. Air Force Academy's course in Colorado Springs hosts more deer than golfers. Two different animals, one with hoofs and one with spikes: one to hit balls, and the other to munch grass. Once when I ripped a drive there, my friend and staunch environmentalist Major Hal Bidlack lurched anxiously down the fairway, flailing his arms in a desperate attempt to alert the deer to the danger of the rapidly approaching scud missile. The deer ignored the major completely and with bemusement stepped calmly aside just out of range of the errant shot. Now I ask you, who was centered in this picture?

Centering training results in persistence and dedication. Witness those foolish fanatics who continue to slosh their way through raging storms in search of the perfect round (or maybe one good shot), while glancing nervously to the sky for signs of lightning, muttering Lee Trevino's famous line, "Even God can't hit a one-iron." Actually, Lee was right. Lightning missed Lee's one-iron and bag altogether and instead nailed the great golfer himself while he was sitting down to wait out a storm. (In fairness, Lee is a bigger target.)

You never get what you expect in golf or centering training. Take holes-in-one. Some golfers have made many in a lifetime of hacking and there are some touring pros who have never made any. I had never even seen one until one unforgettable day while playing with John Denver. The fifteenth hole was a 135-yard par 3 over a lake to an elevated green. The three of us hitting before John had each hit a shot directly at the flag. I couldn't see the green because it was up so high; nonetheless, I was certain of the accuracy of my shot.

I declared, "Probably a gimmie," a tap-in putt for a birdie.

John stepped up, went through his normal ritual featuring a few supersonic windmill practice swings, took one great and long exhalation of breath, hovered ravenlike over his ball, and then launched it far to the right of the pin.

"I hope it stays on the green," the three of us declared. We, in the grand tradition of golf, secretly hoped it had plummeted lemminglike into a ravine down the other side.

As we walked up the hill toward the green, we all did the classic golfers' giraffe gape, stretching our necks to see where our balls were in relation to the pin. Yep, just as I suspected, two were on the green behind the pin, one was probably somewhere in the high grass on the hill behind the green and John's was surely down in the rocky crevasse off the corner of the green. My son, Eri, ever the optimist, happened to glance in the hole while walking past to the other balls.

"Hey, there's one in the hole!" he yells.

Eri pulled out, looked at the markings, and shouted the verdict. "It's J.D.'s ball!"

Now making a hole-in-one is like a grand slam in the World Series, or a three-pointer to win the NBA championship. It's like winning the lottery, having a satori experience, entering Nirvana, or having no wait at your Department of Motor Vehicles office. And witnessing one is a close second. We are talking bragging rights for a lifetime, and a blissful memory etched in the neurons forever. It is divine intervention slam-dunking right in the Golf Devil's face. If I am getting too far out here, just ask John.

What with the jumping around and the high fives and the clubhouse drinks, you would have thought world peace had broken out forever. And when all this subsided, we contemplated my statement that you never get what you expect. John had hit his ball farthest off the mark, but with the hill around the green for it to roll up and come back down, and the particular tilt of the green, it was absolutely the perfect shot. The chance to glimpse such a crack in the cosmic egg is what brings out the hackers on every golf course every weekend in every land.

This past summer, I was warming up on the driving range at my home course when golfing buddy John Black approached. He hovered over me for a few minutes, not saying anything, watching me hit. Now I am no stranger to golf language. John was telling me one of two things, either "Something is seriously wrong with your swing" or "Something amazing just happened in my golf game."

Being rather attached to my swing, I assumed it was the latter.

"So, how you hittin' em?" I asked, which gave him the right to launch into his latest great golf story.

"I'm on the seventeenth hole [a tough 180-yard par 3] with Jesse and two others. We weren't playing all that great. That is, until Jesse launches a shot dead at the pin. It lands on the green, bounces a couple of times, and rolls straight into the cup. None of us could believe it. We've never even seen a hole-in-one. We're going nuts, jumping up and down, wondering if we should continue or go directly to the bar. Anyway, I step up to the tee. Next thing I know, I hit a high fade that drops just over the trap and somehow curls like a heat-seeking missile right towards the hole."

"No! You didn't?" I yelled, alerting the entire driving range.

"Yep!" John beamed. "Two consecutive shots, two holes-in-one! Hell, Jesse didn't even win the hole."

I had to sit down. My brain hurt just contemplating the

112

miraculous nature of such an event. I have a degree in mathematics. What is the probability of that happening? The planet must have been in total alignment, the guys' biorhythms must have been at a lifetime high, they must have accomplished some great humanitarian effort in their past lives, or maybe it was more simple—a secret deal with the Golf Gods. All I know was that true center had struck twice within seconds. To heck with my swing. I picked up my bag and went home to meditate.

And just when I was able to put the whole thing in perspective, I read in a newspaper of a little old lady from Florida in her seventies who got two holes-in-one on consecutive days on the same hole, with the same club, and the same old marked-up golf ball. Sound amazing? Yep. Especially since she was blind.

Another important element of center training is the awareness of the intimate connection between mind and body. Walking and moving with full awareness and a calm mind and body is mindfulness. Golf, like no other sport, demands a similar discipline. To witness the tragic breakdown of that mind-body connection, there is nothing like standing over a four-foot putt on the eighteenth hole with your team counting on you. And all in such a simple activity of rolling a little ball four feet. A simple activity, like sweeping the steps of a monastery. But tell that to the attached, nervous mind with money on the line. As an old Zen master once said, "The mind is of its own place, and of itself can make a heaven of hell, a hell of heaven."

It would seem so simple to just putt the ball four feet, something any golfer could do effectively time after time on the practice green. But out on the course the mind gets cluttered with countless thoughts of failure or success, of punishment or redemption—whatever—when the task is really simple. Chinese Master Po-chang said, "Eat when you are hungry, sleep when you are tired." Po-chang would have drained the putt.

Great golfers know when they are centered. Like breathing, they just swing. Or more accurately, "It" swings.

113

As the famous sixteenth-century Japanese monk Takuan said:

What is most important is to acquire a certain mental attitude known as "immovable wisdom." . . . "Immovable" does not mean to be stiff and heavy and lifeless as a rock or piece of wood. It means the highest degree of mobility with a center which remains immovable. The mind then reaches the highest point of clarity ready to direct its attention anywhere it is needed. . . .

Are you sure Ben Hogan didn't write that? He certainly played with an immovable center. Arms, shoulders, hips, everything else flowed around his center with power and grace.

How golf ever became so strongly established in America is a credit to its mysterious properties. It subverts our do-more, get-busier, frantic lifestyle. Because to play at your optimum level, you must do less, not more—less hurry, less tension, less muscle, less effort, less strokes.

When centered, you realize that companionship is not about who's better. And in golf, you learn quickly that the best companions on the course may not be related to their scoring ability. You can play with anyone regardless of their skill level and have an extraordinary time. Their ability to score well is not the major requirement for companionship. It is the ability to have fun and to be positive and aware that make the best companions. And what many of those golf widows or widowers out there don't realize is that a true golfer can invite a companion along who doesn't even need a club. He or she could just be walking around the course with you, enjoying the moment. Whether you take seventy or a hundred swings, or none at all, it can be a splendid five-mile walk in nature.

And if the score is an issue, golf's handicap system levels the playing field beautifully. And handicaps are in the eye of the beholder. One night over dinner in Boston, Joe Lazaro, the blind golfer who won seven National Blind Golfers Championships, challenged the great Sam Snead to a match and said Sam could name the course and the stakes. Sam did so.

"We'll play at my course," said Sam, shaking hands. "You pick the time."

"Fine," smiled Joe. "How 'bout midnight."

Golf is joy. An old zen verse expresses it well:

> *Oh, this one occurrence*
> *For which would I not be glad to give ten thousand pieces of gold!*
> *A hat is on my head, a bundle around my loins*
> *And on my staff the refreshing breeze and the full moon I carry!*

LEARN TO CENTER THROUGH SPORTS

Once I asked P.G.A. tour player Fred Couples about his weight distribution when he was hitting his short irons. He simply laughed and said, "Heck, I don't know. That's what they write those magazine articles about. All I know is when I'm in balance and when I'm not." Now in sports, balance is paramount, and when it's off, there is immediate feedback. Whether it is a face plant in skiing, or a shank in golf, no one has to tell you. If one of your core purposes for playing sports is to develop center and enhance all aspects of your life, then progress can take place right when the "mistake" is made. Instead of judging yourself harshly, simply accept it completely and move to a centered perspective. It's over, and the only reality you have in truth is this moment. And it is the awareness of the moment, not judgment, that allows you to observe and make distinctions between centered, natural movements versus uncentered, ineffective movements.

Very few of us have taken the opportunity to differentiate between when we are centered and when we are not. We are too afraid to look at and learn from the uncentered moments. Sports, with its immediate feedback system, gives you this opportunity. You don't have to be 100 percent centered. You can be 60 percent centered and 40 percent still caught up in old unworkable patterns. But even a little awareness of center produces progress toward pure center. Without the awareness, you fall into old patterns, repeating behaviors that you have practiced in the past, often inappropriate ones. With centered awareness you can be constantly growing in competency and enjoyment.

To center, relax any tension you feel through deep breathing and focusing on the present moment and the movement. As you do this, you become less outcome-oriented, less focused on the score, the excuses, or the celebration speeches. Instead, you become process-oriented, focused on the ball, the target and your center.

All great athletes go through their ritual, on the tee, or in the starting gate. The rituals may be different for each athlete, but they are repeated precisely the same every time, for a common reason— to get centered so that their movements happen naturally and appropriately.

Success with centering in sports can readily transfer to aspects of life where our self-esteem is not high. For instance, some children have difficulties with math or reading, but are great at soccer or football or some other activity. First acknowledge their talent in those areas. Then, before they start reading, ask them to relive the state they are in when they are playing their sport really well. As they vividly relive those images, and feel the aliveness and power that they possess, their bodies straighten and their minds become alert and relaxed. Now they are ready to read in an aware state, much different than the typical dull state that occurs when they believe they can't do something well. And it works in reverse. Good readers can transfer their alert and quick mental state in reading to increased competency in their sports.

In sports, as in life, it is necessary to strip away the clutter to allow your natural self to emerge. To do this you must Accept What Is (hole-in-one or triple bogey), Learn Through Awareness (be fascinated, not frustrated), and Focus on the Present Moment. With a higher purpose than the score in mind, and persistence and practice at your side, mastery is attainable. More important, so is joy.

Downhill 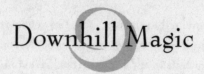Magic

Centered skiing offers a special gift:
Maximum joy and minimum struggle.

I learned skiing as a gung-ho college football player who saw every obstacle as something fun to run into. In 1964, I had my first skiing experience on Whiteface Mountain at Lake Placid, New York. My buddies, already accomplished skiers, had headed up to the top without me. I was still shuffling around like a penguin in my rental ski boots, carrying my poles and skis like a slippery load of firewood, trying to negotiate the door of the ski shop. As I stumbled through, I noticed a couple of ski instructors strolling past with their skis elegantly placed on one shoulder. I quickly got to my feet and looked disdainfully at the door as if it had an architectural defect. I reassembled my gear, assumed the pose of a ski instructor, and walked up to the lift as if I knew what I was doing. You would have thought that if I had that much trouble carrying my skis, I would have been astute enough to take a ski lesson. Nah. I was an indestructible, slightly deranged, nineteen-year-old whose buddies had just gone to the top of the mountain without him.

Nearing the lift, I nonchalantly dropped my skis onto the snow, the way Stein Ericksen would, and gracefully threw one foot onto a ski. Ten minutes later I was still trying to figure out how to connect that foot to the ski with all those cables and straps. Finally, an understanding older lady who probably had a teenage alien being of her own helped me to get strapped in and ready to go. I resumed my ultracool look, and began to glide over to the lift. It was as if I had suddenly stepped on a treadmill running at full speed. I countered the backwards sliding with about ten fast steps at sprinter speed, barely staying in the same place, before accomplishing my first face plant. I struggled to my feet quickly to avoid being noticed by the many snickering people around me and began to fiddle with my bindings as if *that* were the culprit. This absurd diversion did allow me to catch a peek at how others could move so easily. Eventually, I recognized the usefulness of my ski poles and pushed my way to the chair lift.

What an ingenious device! A chair came whipping around the corner, knocked my legs out from under me, and flipped me backward onto the seat. In football a clip like that would have resulted in a fifteen-yard penalty. Off I went, clenching a metal bar with one hand and some guy's leg with the other.

Getting onto the chairlift as a beginner may have been a lesson in survival. Getting off was one in sheer terror. It's amazing how time speeds up when you're confused. I watched my chair speeding toward what appeared to my beginner's eye to be the ramp of an Olympic ski jump. Simultaneously, I tried to grab my poles, put my skis in reasonably parallel form in front of me, and ready my body for impact. Just as I was catapulted from my chair at the top of the ramp, I noticed, splayed at the bottom of the ramp, a very large woman in very small stretch pants. What's the etiquette at a time like this? I braced myself for the collision, trying to avoid the wide target on a narrow runway, ignoring the old hang-glider adage, "Don't look where you don't want to land."

119

9

Behind us the chair kept unloading more wide-eye kamikazes onto the ramp, which increased the pileup, featuring me and my newly intimate large friend in the very small stretch pants. Finally, his sadistic tendencies satiated, the lift operator stopped the lift and began to unstack the bodies. The fact that we were all uninjured and laughing was a great statement of humanity. The lift systems have gotten safer since the early sixties, and they're not nearly as much fun.

The top of Whiteface Mountain on an icy day is beginner's hell. I became desperately connected to the mountain. One part or another of my anatomy embraced it with every attempted turn. But, hey! I was a strong, tough football player who didn't mind taking a few shots. The occasional cheering from the chairlift above at my high-speed wipeouts made up for any permanent damage I was doing to my life-support system. I decided that this was the best contact sport ever created. I knew then that I would become a skier.

Years later, when I moved to Aspen, I was still under the impression that skiing was like a war between me and the mountain. It was a military campaign, and the best strategy was a blitzing offense—attack and never give an inch. And for a while it worked. But only for the same reasons that countries send people aged eighteen to twenty-five to fight their battles. They're young, crazy, and consider themselves immortal. Trees, steeps, bumps, and cliffs—these were my battlegrounds on the ski mountain. And always, no matter how good I thought I was getting, there was always a patch of ice that would bring me back to a state of humility. Even chairlifts, years after my inauspicious beginning, continued to get the best of me.

120

It was one of the finest season openings ever on Thanksgiving Day, circa 1970, in Snowmass. About two feet of fresh new powder had fallen the previous two days, with more on the way. A few fanatic buddies and I were at the lift forty-five minutes early so we would be the ones to catch the first chair of the new season. To our dismay there were about twenty rabid folks ahead of us. Catching that first chair was always a distinguished honor to a true ski bum, but even the eleventh chair assured us of an untracked powder beginning.

On powder mornings the ride up is a ritual. While cleaning your goggles and fixing your neck gaiter, you first swap sagas detailing the arduous effort to get there that early. Then the great debate begins.

"This could be the greatest day yet. I bet there's eighteen inches already."

"Nah. Remember that dump this time two years ago? Now *that* was awesome!"

"Heck, that was nothing compared to December of 'sixty-six."

It's uncanny how deadly accurate the brain is when it comes to recalling the millimeters of snow depth on powder days or the jersey number of any sports figure since World War II. Especially when such genius comes from the same people who can't remember the first two out of three items he was supposed to pick up at the grocery store (the third item being the cookies).

But eventually the chairlift debate shifted to which runs to ski—a strategically paramount issue if we were to maximize the amount of untracked powder. Since some of my friends were in the chairs behind me, I was turned around as far as I could to hear their ideas. The next thing I heard was the sound of my chair companion, Bruce, getting off the lift. By the time I turned back around, I was five feet past the off-ramp and heading to the big bull wheel, where the chairlift reverses direction and heads downhill, traditionally riderless. To add to my humiliation, I had to pass over the heads of ten ski patrolmen who were standing at the bottom of the ramp to greet the first skiers of the year. With eyes rolled to the heavens, they shook their heads, wondering who was dumb enough not to get off the lift. I pulled my

9

hat and goggles down to hide my identity as the vibrating chair clanged around the wheel before its return trip to the ramp. There the lift operator stopped the chair so that I could descend and take my final bows.

Skiing. Why do we call it that? Did some ancient Scandinavian standing on two pine boards hear that sound while plummeting down a glacier? Or is it a divinely ordained onomatopoeia? The word "skiing" does sound like the noise made by sharp edges on ice. If our ancient Scandinavian friend had been less proficient, maybe we would be calling it "schrapping" today. But then, if deep powder had been the condition, "whooshing" about would be a regular winter activity. Having a great pair of "whooshes" has a ring to it, doesn't it? All of which is better than naming it after the sounds that many beginners make, "Oh sh—!"

The worst blizzards are the best times to ski if you are a fanatic, because there are very few people around. Kind of the same reason so few surf during a hurricane. On one such day, where we couldn't see beyond our ski tips, my buddies and I were crashing down through eighteen inches of fresh powder, whoopin' and hollerin' with each turn. I was whooshing down a steep line in the trees. When the visibility is poor, the woods allow you to see the terrain much better. The downside is that there is much less of it. The idea here is not really to "ski in the trees" but to ski the space between them. Suddenly, I found myself rocketing out of the good visibility of the woods into a treeless whiteout. Almost immediately I felt my body lurch forward as my tips rammed into a concealed dip. And, just as immediately, I was thrown back as my skis exploded over the top of the dip. I heard my lower leg snap. The amazing thing was that I was still standing. I stood there long enough for my howling buddies to catch up, and let out the typical cheers that always follow a great run. Then I told them I had just broken my leg.

"What are you talking about?" Bruce laughed. "You never fell."

"Maybe if I had, I wouldn't have this problem." They helped me sit carefully in the snow and called for the ski patrol.

Lying in the hospital while the doctor placed a cast on my leg, I happened to catch a reflection of my image in a window to my left. I saw a young man with a leg cast in a good deal of pain. Then the image transformed into me at younger ages, with different injuries. Seven years old with my left elbow in a cast suspended by a hook above the hospital bed. Twelve years old with face and head taped with stitches. It was like a slide show—collarbone, ankle, finger, back, knee, other knee. Different ages, different activities, same dumb kid. What did I need to learn? How many more years of abuse before I could only sit in a chair and stare at the floor?

I began to consider the pattern. In each accident I had been unaware and uncentered. I could recall the moment of injury but not the moment *before* injury. Could these accidents have been eliminated with awareness training, centering training?

In skiing, the mountain is much bigger than we are. (Actually, they are bigger even if you are not skiing.) The hill isn't an opposing linebacker or street mugger. All of our physical strength means nothing to a tree or boulder or a slab of ice. There's really nothing to conquer, no legitimate objective way to measure who won and who lost. Fighting a mountain is like grabbing an ocean wave. Grab as you like, it disappears in your hand. The wave doesn't care. The mountain doesn't fight. It doesn't have to. It just is.

One week later I was back on the mountain with one leg in a cast and the other on a ski, ready to go. The doctor hadn't told me I *couldn't* ski with the cast on, so why not? Nowadays there are wonderful disabled skier programs, which feature little skis that you can attach to ski poles for added balance and support. But back then I was playing a whole new game; I had to treat myself and the mountain differently. We would have to be danc-

123

9

ing partners. It was here—skiing on just one leg—that I began actively to practice in skiing something I had been exploring in the martial arts—the concept of centering.

I pushed off, all my weight on my good left leg. I made a pretty nice natural turn to my right. But when I attempted to go left (or to turn on the outside edge of my ski), I fell. I got up again and pushed off, but this time I was more aware of my natural center—the area between my hips. Over a series of wipeouts I found that if I maintained a relaxed awareness of center at a point a couple of inches below my navel and visualized energy flowing out from center through my head, arms, and legs, I could ski a turn or two before crashing. I was unifying myself (literally "bonding") with the mountain and the environment around me. Right before falling I'd start noticing that I could actively feel my loss of center and connection. I would stand back up and consciously extend energy from my center down the hill to a specific location several turns away. The more I could feel the dynamic connection between center and where I was heading, the more effective I would be at arriving there, still standing. Turn by turn, I began to lengthen the distance traveled.

Before long I had such a heightened sensitivity to my center that turning ceased to be a problem. Instead, leg cramps, or more precisely "leg cramp," became the issue. I would ski for a hundred yards or so and have to pull up, completely exhausted. Then I noticed that I was holding my leg in semi-isometric contraction for the entire time. I began to switch metaphors, and think of my leg as fluid and flowing. As I worked with this metaphor, I noticed not only a reduction of the rigidity and exhaustion in my leg, but also a heightened sensitivity to my ski and its connection to the snow. I felt like I was barefoot on the grass, feeling everything. To make an outside turn (to the left of my good left leg) I could roll the ski over from inside edge to outside and feel the connection, stability, and power. Wow. I had felt none of this during the previous years of mountain battles. And that was on two legs.

Within a month I could ski the whole mountain on one leg—black diamond runs, mogul fields, trees, you name it. And I was skiing better technically than I had been on two legs. I would occasionally get cocky about my new prowess, lose my awareness, and go from stardom to a yard sale, my ski poles, hat, and goggles scattered everywhere. But instead of the old upset and judgment, I could now observe *when* it happened and *why*. I had a newfound fascination with outcome, rather than frustration over failure. Of course, I was not totally void of old patterns. During one particular ego-driven skirmish, I bounced so hard on a mogul that my cast broke in half and I had to return to the hospital for a new fitting. But the cast had done its job, and the leg had not been damaged further. My doctor had been unaware of my skiing. His original "no worry" attitude had referred to simply walking around and general activities. But by that time I was nearly healed anyway, both in leg and, in an important new way, in spirit.

I began to commit myself more fully to the art of centering. I became even more devoted to aikido. I started to understand the nature of ki, or energy, and our unlimited potential to extend it outward to the environment around us. And it was the direct application of the principles of aikido (relaxation, power, balance, gravity) to skiing that became the basis of our annual Magic of Skiing seminars, taught each year in Aspen and sponsored by the Aspen Ski Company.

The snow war had ended. A new dance had begun. The focus was now, quite simply, creating maximum joy with minimum effort while sliding down a snowy mountain. A ski affair can blossom into a committed relationship. As in any long-term relationship, it's constantly changing and challenging. It's sometimes smooth, sometimes bumpy, often intense and fast, occasionally gradual and soothing. There are hard spots that leave us bruised and sore, in contrast to those moments of ecstasy when it's deep and soft.

When we were kids, we didn't have to remind ourselves that sliding down a mountain was all play and learning. Getting too serious about how you looked, at the expense of how you felt, was silly. Juxtapose a seven-year-old at warp speed blazing past a barely moving adult hunched over in a rigid, held snowplow position. The youngster is more on track. He understands that the whole idea is to slide downhill, not to stay stuck in one place on the mountain. We adults tend to approach the principles of gravity, mass, and momentum as intellectual concepts. When we are on two slick boards, facing downhill, we are supposed to experience those principles, not fight them. But, hey, I understand. It's a little scary to the middle-aged adult with more scar tissue and much farther to fall then some three-and-a-half-foot-tall pre-adolescent missile. But, as adults we need to support each other in recapturing the fun of childhood, the joy of play.

Little kids are constantly reminding us what skiing's really about. Forget about ski fashion, technically precise equipment, and the antifog spray for your goggles. Kids, in fact, forget almost everything but the essence—sliding down a mountain on white stuff. If the average adult skier has a boot a little too loose or a tad too tight, then the whine begins. The only thing holding them back from an unsurpassed Olympic performance is the "jerk" who sold them their boots. (The one who bought them is apparently off the hook.)

I was teaching a group of five-year-olds one day. "Teaching" means jump-the-bumps with different animal sounds on the way down and belting out "Little Bunny Foo-Foo" on the chairlift riding back up. On one particular "Big Bear" jump, a little pigtailed munchkin came flying off the lip making perfect *reedeep* frog sounds. The next thing I knew, two skis complete with boots attached were racing toward me in perfect parallel, but there was no skier! Just a ghost downhiller whizzing past me and disappearing into the trees below. I looked back uphill and there was the little girl, on her back with her stockinged feet raised to the heavens, focusing happily on catching snowflakes with her tongue. Are we having fun or what?

Some of us remember how magical snow was when we were children. The clear, clean taste of the flakes on our tongues, the fantastic crystalline patterns they formed as they landed on our gloves. The excitement of waking up to big heavy flakes floating to earth, creating a blanket of wonder and fun. The early morning radio stations announcing the closing of school, the ringing of the telephone as wide-eyed friends planned their day of sledding, snowman building, and snowball fights. And the endless hours of just jumping, falling, and laughing in the deep white playground, barely able to stand with the weight of the four or five layers of clothing our moms had insisted that we wear. Then into the house frozen and dripping wet, to dry out and drink hot chocolate while our clothes tumbled in the dryer in preparation for the next assault.

And, oh, that Flexible Flyer! That wonderful Christmas sled—the one that had been dry-docked all summer in the corner of the basement, now ready for action! The thrill of careening down a kid-made luge run with two or three buddies piled on top screaming in our ears as we sped toward the dreaded jump that the big kids had made, closing our eyes at the last minute as the inevitable blizzard of snow consumed our faces and flew down our backs and into that space where pant legs and boots never meet. Then the look of delight at the debris of buddies strewn left and right, declaring *that* run to be the best run ever, and then pulling each other up to hurry to catch one more run before it was time to go in.

Too many of us have lost touch with that child-like wonder, possibly out of frustration and fear. Many of us have quit skiing, injured or discouraged from fighting the mountain rather than dancing with it. Skiing is a time to let go of our adult dilemmas and enjoy gliding freely down snow-covered mountains. And technology has made it so much easier to play—lightweight clothing that can keep us both dry and warm, high-speed lifts that can swoop us up thousands of feet in minutes, and high-tech equipment and highly qualified coaches that can support us in standing up on two feet and safely skiing down the white stuff with more joy and control than ever before. And the hot chocolate still comes with marshmallows.

The need to center in skiing is never-ending. Once ski coach Tom Eckstein and I were videotaping a group of expert skiers on a steep run on Aspen Mountain one sunny day. Tom, entrusted with my video camera with all the goodies, was zooming in on one of our students, who was making quick, short radius turns toward us. I was standing right behind Tom, narrating.

The footage recorded as follows:

"Wow! Look at Christy making some great turns down North Star. Her skis are moving very fast, but notice how she remains in good speed control by completing her turns and making consistent radius turns. Excellent. She is . . . She's . . . Tom! *Aggg-h-hh!!!*" (Video shots of spinning trees, turning sky, then total darkness.)

Regrettably, my camera was in two pieces. But thankfully, Tom, Christy, and I were in three pieces, although twisted, sore, and intertwined.

On the other hand, being just a little bit more centered can make all the difference. I was participating in a clinic of ski pros on a very icy day on Aspen Mountain. Eleven of us were standing and listening intently to the clinic leader situated below us. I happened to be standing at the end of the line and thus farther uphill than the rest. Suddenly, I had an intense feeling of energy coming from uphill, directly behind me. I turned just in time to see a skier moving at a highly unadvisable speed, about to fall face first a few feet above me. It was like a scuba diver turning just in time to see a great white shark speeding in for the kill. No time to think. The next thing I knew, I had, with a shout, jumped straight up in the air. Miraculously, he flew right under my skis and bowled down the entire rest of the group below me. Hollers, ski poles, and curses flew. It was a perfect strike: ten pros laid out in piles along the mountain, uninjured but livid. The human bowling ball was a high school ski racer who must have wished he had otter-slid the final two miles down the mountain, boarded a bus, and gone home. He did get his ski pass suspended for his recklessness, but some of the pros wanted his scalp too. Little did they know we already had it: directly below me on the snow was a big tuft of black hair. His head had come so close to my ski edges that, as he slid under me, he left a good portion of his mane behind. It gave "hair-raising moments" a new meaning.

And it isn't only the expert who finds the true Magic. Take, for instance, one beloved student named Maggie. She was approaching fifty but had never skied before, not just because of her fear, but because, as she cheerfully says, "I can hardly stand up on dry ground, much less on two sliding pieces of wood."

Buttermilk Mountain in Aspen is ideally suited for someone like Maggie. There is a wide flat area to begin walking and sliding. And there is a beginner's chairlift that takes you to Panda Peak, a run that's ideal for getting comfortable with turning, stopping, and letting the skis run straight. And, easiest of all, there was Tipi Hill, leveled for very young children, with a snowcat that pulls them slowly up a slope that's so gradual you can't see the grade unless you squint.

This is where Maggie began her training.

This big woman with a gentle heart was terrified. But she drew her courage from the three-year-olds around her. Together

129

they held on to the snowcat for the slow ride up the "hill."

Maggie found more than skiing. She found the present moment. Some people progress from beginner to expert runs in a few days. But none possess more Magic than Maggie. A week later you *could* find Maggie turning and stopping at will (er, *mostly* at will). But where *would* you find her? Still with the preschoolers, laughing and singing their way up and down Tipi Hill.

> *If the secret is disclosed, it will be so simple*
> *that everyone may get a good laugh.*

—*CHANG PO-TUAN*

CHOOSE BELIEFS THAT WORK

Would you like to enjoy yourself more in some activity? It's not a certain performance or skill level that holds the real key to enjoyment. It's about taking charge of your beliefs.

When I first started teaching skiing, I noticed that each of my students had a different "guideline" about his or her skiing. Some had a certain crazed look in their eyes when the talk turned to an approaching storm and the possibility of deep powder. The bigger the whiteout, the happier they became. In fact, anytime they had an opportunity to be on the mountain, they were pumped up and ready to go, whether the conditions were ice, crud, cement, occasional rocky spots, or perfect powder. Author Ken Blanchard summed it up the best, "Anytime I'm skiing, it's a great day."

But others did not share this enthusiasm. They made comments like "I only feel good about skiing when it's warm and the sun is out." Or "I feel good about skiing when the snow is hard-packed and groomed."

I began to observe how our beliefs literally made the difference between a "gung-ho" ski nut, constantly improving, and the "terminal intermediate," who had not progressed in years. The avid skier felt challenge, opportunity, and enthusiasm in all conditions. Weather was not a controlling factor on his or her ability to enjoy and feel good. But in the terminal intermediate's belief, the quality of feeling was often dependent upon weather or snow conditions, neither of which the skier could control.

Along with the weather and snow conditions, here were some other disempowering conditions for feeling good while skiing:

"When I feel like I'm one of the best skiers in the group."

"When my friends (and particularly my instructor) like the way I ski."

"When I don't fall down or screw up."

"When I'm technically improving everyday."

"When everybody in my group is happy."

In each of these, the power for personal enjoyment was given to something external. It was dependent upon something beyond their control: someone else's opinion or mood, or an unrealistic level of proficiency, or nothing but perfect weather. No wonder the end result was a less enthusiastic, lethargic attitude toward skiing. With disempowering edicts like these, activities you start out loving will eventually be cast aside because they become work and struggle.

Now consider the answers the ski fanatics give when I ask, "When do *you* feel good about skiing?"

"When I'm learning something."

"When I'm feeling my center and balance and my connection to the skis and snow."

"When I let go of my judgments about my technique as compared with someone else's."

"When I embrace my emotions and process my fears rather than get paralyzed by them."

"When I'm breathing that good clean mountain air and remembering how grateful I am to be here."

131

9

And as Magic of Skiing coach Weems Westfeldt says with a gleam, stepping into his bindings, "When I hear 'the click'!"

Is there a difference in these? You bet. Each one places the choice of feeling good about yourself upon you. You have the control and power each moment to breathe, get centered, let go, and learn for the sheer joy of it. Take a good hard look at your disempowering rules and change them to ones you can control. Whether you're going skiing, schrapping, whooshing, or anywhere, choose beliefs that work.

It's About Time

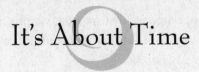

What happens to time
when we ride the light?

My trouble with Time began as a child when my parents were never on time. They were always early. Left to my own internal timepiece, I would have meandered through the day quite happily, being prompt only to those events that seemed relevant, and not at all to others. I know my parents and teachers were just doing their best to instill "responsibility" in me, yet with each year, from school days to church, the time crunch pressed more tightly. Only during the more divinely inspired events would Time and I commune. Never once was I late for a Sunday afternoon touch football game.

Through *no* fault of my own, you understand (sympathy music starts about here), I had fallen victim to that acute disease "time anxiety." Time became the dragon breathing down my neck, the devil robbing me of my peace, the clock on the scoreboard knocking me out of the "zone." Maybe soon this highly contagious disease will be isolated in a researcher's test tube, and a subsequent vaccine will eliminate this virus and the guilt cruelly heaped upon poor, unsuspecting victims like myself. I'm a victim, I tell you! But until that fortuitous day, time anxiety remains a very real disability.

Folks who haven't contracted the disease probably can't relate to what I'm saying. They have sufficient natural antibodies to transform Time into a reliable friend offering structure and certainty to their lives. But for people like me, it just ain't so.

Take travel, for example, which I do a lot of. Planes don't wait. The old battle with Time becomes high drama. Let's say I have a flight in midafternoon. I start the day "on time" and focused, but through either serendipitous happenings or karmic predicaments, I'm inevitably sprinting to catch my plane.

Ironically, I've learned to be comfortable in my dysfunctional relationship with Time. I can accept weaving through traffic in taxis, glancing at my watch, watching for any critical delays of precious seconds, adrenaline flowing, jumping out at curbside, sprinting down the concourse, collapsing into my seat for **the win!** I'm practically undefeated in the great plane race.

Although I have become comfortable in the pressurized rush to the airport, I notice that it cripples my travel companions. It's the subtle things, like when they shout obscenities or sweat profusely, that convince me I should try to break my habit. But wanting to change old behaviors and actually changing them are two different things.

I have tried programming my subconscious with the lyrics of one of my Rolling Stones favorites, *"T-i-i-ime is on my side. Yes it is."* But one of the great benefits of music is that just when you think your middle-aged brain cells are failing, an old rock-and-roll tune can stimulate total recall. So, along with my positive programming, my neurons serve up images of high school days, lying on my bed on a very early Sunday morning after a very late Saturday night. The roar of the lawn mower cranking up below my window. An even crankier father mumbling just loudly enough to reach my pillow, "Well, if he's not going to do his job, I'll have to do it for him."

A few years ago I was visiting my parents at their home in Florida. I had a few days off before another round of seminars. Just lie around, eat, and play golf. But as my departure day approached, Time turned into Mr. Hyde. Or was it my father who did? When for the umpteenth time (parents are good at "umpteenth") my dad inquired about the time of my upcoming flight, I began to get that crazy feeling again, that I was back in high school on a Saturday night trying to negotiate a new curfew without creating a war.

I had a 10 A.M. flight from Tampa to Rochester, New York. Tampa was only an hour's drive from my parents' home, and Dad wanted me to leave at 7 A.M. That, I judged, was outrageous. After several small skirmishes, both of us became closed down and grumpy, each in our own way—sudden interest in the newspaper, gruffness, quick answers and fiercer opinions about any topic. But once I came up from the mud long enough to breathe, I began to recognize these old patterns. Over a "Pass the mayonnaise" opportunity at lunch, I responded with, "You know, I think that seven o'clock would be fine. I'll be ready." There. I had done it. Immediately, the scenery brightened. And Dad's response? "Oh, I think seven-thirty will give us plenty of time."

That evening, before bedtime, I did the unusual. I mentally ran through the familiar pattern of feeling rushed and hurried by good old Dad. In the morning he would be hanging around waiting, watching me pack, checking his watch. I planned every action and detail in advance so that I would be ready to go at 7:15 A.M.

In the morning I was geared up for success. It wasn't easy, given my talent for dawdling. It's amazing how mesmerizing a magazine article can be when you're in the john, or how a sudden revelation about your golf swing can keep you captive in the shower. But each time I heroically brought myself back to the mission, and with fifteen minutes to spare I was ready to go. My father had to hustle to catch up.

We drove off at seven-twenty sharp, two happy travelers. That is, until we got to the Tampa freeway system, where my father took his traditional wrong turn. Several mistakes later, after he had cursed every traffic light, every motorist (and their bumper stickers), highway engineers in general and the secretary of transportation in particular, we limped our way into the Tampa airport. Still, we were there at 8:45 A.M., *way* ahead of the ten o'clock departure.

"It's good we left early. Otherwise, we barely would have made it," Dad said proudly.

Ah. But, if we had left an hour later, and I had driven, wouldn't we have been here in more than enough time? Good question. But only a fool would pose it.

Instead, I looked at my dad fondly. As much as we fought about time, the old guy was right-on about a lot of other things. All the modern and scientific high-tech ideas about health and fitness, diet and longevity, didn't stand up to the living example of this feisty and vitally alive man of ninety wondering "What's for dessert?" He never missed a dessert and he never missed being early (except for his death which, given statistics on U.S. males, he is late for already).

Dad was now looking at his watch, concerned about my being on time to check my bags. "Relax, Dad," I laughed. "I'm only going to New York. I'm not going to Iraq." Earlier in the week this could have created another war, but Dad was wise enough to remember that old family principle of always parting congenially.

"Well, have a good trip," he replied lovingly.

I responded with a big hug, embarrassing him as usual, handshakes being far more suitable to his generation. (You never heard John Wayne say "I love you." When I first got up the courage to utter such alien words to my dad, the best he could muster was "Yeah, you too.")

Dad drove off and I walked to the ticket counter. I was encouraged with my progress in dealing with my old nemesis, Time. Here I was, with an entire *hour and a quarter* to relax. *"Time is on my side. Yes it is."*

Now what should I do? Should I read a novel or, better yet, write one? Or make those overdue phone calls to old friends? Or do nothing and just watch the people? All the things I wished I had time for when I had been running behind. And now I finally had the time! But the novel looked boring, my imagination withered under the weight of my pen, my old friends and I would probably make awkward small talk, and the people I was watching, instead of "doing" their life at the moment were simply spectating like me, putting their life on hold until they got to their destinations. This newfound time was not as easy to deal with as I thought. If I was going to get comfortable with this being-early business, I was going to need to practice.

So I fell asleep.

"We will begin early boarding on United Flight 703 to Philadelphia and on to Rochester," came the announcement.

As I took my seat on the plane, I closed my eyes to meditate.

"I need to get by you to my seat."

The loud demand startled me. I looked up at a thin, anxious beak chirping above me. A large bird of a woman, tall, sharp, and angular, was pointing to the window seat next to me. My enraptured Audubon Society look was no doubt disconcerting. She dropped her handbag in the aisle, and with one predator swoop scooped it up while simultaneously fluttering past me to her new perch. Strange species indeed. A stern, purposeful stare when I caught her eye kept me from further inquiry. Fear of extinction, I assumed, so I slipped back into meditation.

137

"This is the captain speaking." I was brought to attention by the intercom.

"I'm sorry to inform you that this flight has been delayed due to severe thunderstorms. You are free to deplane if you would like. We will inform you as new information becomes available."

I glanced at my watch. I'd been at the airport an hour and a half already. I had left my parents' home many hours ago. The skill of hurrying I had learned very well. The lesson of patience was not quite as well honed. Hmm . . . I drifted off into a light stupor contemplating all the things I would have accomplished had I started in my normal late mode. I could have spent more time lounging in bed, worked out, taken a long shower . . . Sometimes being right is fun.

I passed another hour in my seat, listening to the captain's periodic announcements. I became more righteous with each delay.

"I'm sorry to inform you that our flight will be delayed another thirty minutes."

I looked at my watch. I had been sitting in my seat for well over an hour and we were still parked at the gate. I decided to stretch my legs with a little stroll, make a quick phone call, and maybe grab a snack. As I entered the terminal, I glanced at my watch. The new, prudent me decided that I should take only fifteen minutes. I noticed that the bank of phones across from the gate were all in use, with several people queued up in wait. I walked down two gates before coming to an open phone. I called my assistant Judy, who was organizing the workshop in Rochester. I mentioned the weather delay and assured her not to worry.

"I'm glad that you took an early flight out." She paused. "It's not like you."

"That's because it wasn't the early flight. It was the only flight," I replied. "See you soon!"

I hung up and went to the rest room. After a few minutes I returned to the concourse. Fifteen minutes had passed. Since I had time to spare, I proceeded leisurely to the gate. About halfway there I noticed that there were no people at the phones and in fact there were no longer any people milling around at the boarding area.

There's no way, came the panicked thought. No way. I'm certain he said thirty minutes.

I began to walk more quickly, on the lookout for some people, some sign, any sign that I was just paranoid. But I somehow knew the nightmare was true and began running to the gate. As I came into view of the actual gate door, I knew. It was shut. I frantically ran to the window. My airplane was taxiing to the runway, only yards away from the gate. I looked around the terminal. No one at the counter, only a few people standing at an adjacent gate.

And then, I did that strange thing that emerges out of the panic state. I began to shout at the airplane.

"No! Come back! It hasn't been a half hour. You can't do this."

The plane did not respond.

"What the hell is going on here?"

I demanded justice to descend from the heavens. Or at least from the guy reading the newspaper and pretending not to hear me.

It's fascinating to be conscious enough to witness embarrassing yourself and then stupid enough to continue to do so. It's always easier to pull this feat off anonymously. Rush-hour traffic is an ideal place to watch the phenomenon on a daily basis. People yelling and venting their inner wrath upon other equally off-centered crazies, all of whom are protected by layers of metal. Although we have all practiced such behaviors on the highway, it takes another level of uncenteredness to perform them in an airport terminal. There I was unleashing a litany of abuse on not simply the airline, but on big business, my parents, Father Time, all religions and governments, and my chewing gum that had lost its flavor. Once I became aware of my embarrassing behavior, I did another curious thing. Instead of giving it up, I began to wallow in it and increase the embarrassment. It's the strange theory that says that once you've revealed yourself for the unbalanced person that you are, then you can really show them how unglued you can be.

I turned and raced defiantly down the concourse to the next gate, to the first airline employee I could find, so I could unload my righteous indignation, hopefully moving her to tears and rapid action. Wrong. She simply delivered a detached "I'm sorry" and sent me to Customer Service. Customer Service shrugged off my wild-eyed laments and merely stated that the flight options were nonexistent on their airline, but there was a chance I could catch another airline to Atlanta, then Washington, and eventually Rochester by midnight. But when they asked to see my ticket, another shock hit me. I had left everything on the airplane seat—tickets, coat, money, dignity—everything that was my life-support kit and connection to reality. I caught a vivid image of the empty airplane seat with all my personal belongings being scrutinized by the discerning eye of the bird lady. I could almost hear her squawking, "He hasn't come back. Must be some kind of terrorist."

Eventually, I ended up in the terminal manager's office. The anger and outrage had subsided, with naked resignation in its stead. Slowly, my long-lost center returned. Somehow I began to realize that my little dilemma was not quite critical enough to force the airline to designate a DC-10 for my own personal use. Nor was the president of the United States likely to send *Air Force One* down to get me. The more important challenge was to get this manager to understand that although I had no money and no ticket, simply the clothes on my back, that I had indeed been on the plane that I had missed. And that I had to get to a city today that they didn't fly to until tomorrow.

I breathed deeply from center, "I know you're probably very

busy, but I wonder if you would take a few minutes to help me out of this big dilemma that I've gotten into?"

It was long past midnight when I crawled into Rochester via other airlines and cities. As I stood in the baggage claim office negotiating with the claims person to do a search for my personal belongings that I discovered later had been confiscated by dubious airport officials in Philadelphia, I knew one thing for certain: the only plane I had ever been really early for, I had missed.

After due consideration I concluded that missing-the-plane-I-had-been-early-for must have been an aberration, and that the practice of being early was still something I would benefit from. I decided to retest the theory when I entered the America's Uphill. This demented event happens every March in Aspen. A few hundred slightly deranged folks gather at the base of Aspen Mountain at 7 A.M. for a shotgun-start race to the top (about three miles straight uphill). You equip yourself for one of several categories: lightweight racing skis, telemark skis (cross-country), "heavy metal" mountaineering skis, or snowshoes. Each year I lie myself into thinking that I'll just take my time and not concern myself with results. Every year I think of it as a community gathering, a neighborly stroll up the mountain with no pressure. But when the adrenaline surge rushes through my system at the sound of the gun, I blast out of the gate at gut-twisting speed, wheezing and gasping my way to a personal record, feeling somehow great and lousy all at the same time.

"No one really cares about your time," participants tell one another the week before, as they secretively research the latest finding on carbo-loading. But as the week progresses, the coals of competition glow hotter. There I was in my mid-forties with one eye focused on peace of mind and the other on my anaerobic threshold. Once again my ego needed to prove itself worthy by getting somewhere within a certain range of minutes. "What happened to the fun community event?" I asked myself as my stomach churned with fear that my equipment wasn't high-tech enough for a decent performance. In self-defense I planned my escape route. Sore knee, tight groin, a strategically placed little cough. But there was no escaping, so I began to consider the possibility of repatterning all of this self-inflicted stress. Instead of the usual time-driven anxiety of running around the morning of the race getting my equipment together, barely getting into line before the gun, I decided on surprising old Father Time with the "new" me. I planned on being fully prepared and ready at the starting line about fifteen minutes *before* the gun.

No hassle, no worry, no clock ticktocking away at my stomach lining. With great discipline I actually pulled off this massive change in my old pattern. Heaven forbid, but I even prepared the latest training meal recipe the night before. By morning I had so much extra time I invited my wife, Cathy, and our one-year-old black Labrador puppy, Maggie, to walk with me to the race. The world looked different with all this free time. There were only about fifty racers present when we got there. Gone was the normal jockeying for position that would occur among the hundreds who would be arriving minutes later. So why was I so uncomfortable?

The thing about old patterns is that you're comfortable in them. They may be kicking the hell out of you in terms of the quality of life, but at least you are at ease with the familiarity of the pain. It's like throwing your back out. The one position that feels good looks awkward and throws everything else out of whack. Then something else goes out because of the twisted compensation, and before long you are walking around with your head bent in one direction and your hips in another. Totally dysfunctional. But at least you feel best in that gnarled position. And if you make an adjustment toward a more aligned state by straightening the head and the hip, the discomfort of

142

doing so shows up immediately. And, it is precisely the discomfort of the more balanced state that we use as a justification for returning to the old familiar twisted one.

Standing in the front row with ten minutes to spare put me in discomfort immediately. First, my mind actually had the time to think, not the normal state when I'm scurrying about just to make the starting gate. I had a new worry with each thought: equipment, tight groin, race strategy. I realized that it was 6:45 A.M. and the temperature was twenty degrees and I was standing there in tights and a light windbreaker. Cathy noticed my concern and offered me her coat, a full-length down parka. What a great idea. I could stay warm right up to seconds before the gun and just throw it to the side when ready. It was too snug and the peach color definitely wasn't me, but the warmth was appreciated. I looked lovingly over at Cathy, shivering loyally in my light windbreaker. I felt no guilt.

Within minutes the hustling and bustling of the hundreds of racers began. I was mesmerized by the crowd from my new perspective at the front of the line, and I turned around to watch them jostling for position. I neglected to see the starter appear at the other end of the line. The noise of conversation, the clanging of skis and boots, and my own thoughts about a triumphant race strategy actually drowned out his quick welcome and even quicker countdown. There I was, right in front, so early, so ahead of the game, discussing the weather with the person in back of me, when the starting gun sounded.

Waves of skiers came crushing down upon me as I stood paralyzed in my full-length peach parka. Two full rows whizzed past me before I stuck my poles in the snow and threw the parka off my shoulders in one grand movement. To no avail. Both sleeves were stuck on my forearms. I tried to pull it off in reverse. It only tightened the hold of the sleeves on my arms. More rows of stampeding skiers passed. I yelled to Cathy. She weaved through the rush-hour crush of skiers to get to me. She

143

began to yank at the coat in an effort to help. I tried to assist by skiing away with my forearms behind. Meanwhile, Maggie, at that aggressive puppy age, recognized this as a massive game of tug-of-war. She leaped up, bit the sleeve of the parka and started yanking it—and me—in an entirely new direction. The last row of skiers passed, laughing hysterically at my plight. With dog on one arm and Cathy on the other, I tried frantically to ski up the mountain, hoping to pull my arms free of them both. Finally, one arm popped loose and I was able to shake my iron-jawed dog off the other as Cathy ran back for my poles. I had battled my way twenty yards up the slope during the tug-of-war. The last wave of humanity was fifty yards ahead, with the guys in the front row two hundred yards or more, fading rapidly in the distance. I was out of breath, full of sweat and furious. Cathy and the other spectators were rolling with laughter.

Like a wild-eyed thief with a guard dog on his pants, I caught up with the pokey last row of skiers. I was fully anaerobic, fire in my lungs, and anger in my gut. Only 2.9 miles left to go—straight uphill.

"At this rate," I coughed, "I'll pass out with two miles left." I looked through my sweat at the back row of skiers that I had caught up with. They were chatting about sleeping bags! Here I was wheezing my way through strain and struggle toward the very vindication of my soul, and they had the audacity to be having a chat about the warmth/weight ratio of down versus synthetic fiber. Didn't they know this was *a Race!?* Somehow the contradiction of my cursing and their chatting sunk in. I laughed. I breathed deep and full from my center rather than from my chest. I looked over at my two skinny companions.

"Did you notice that guy back there in a pink parka?" I asked.

"Yeah. The one with the dog hanging on? Unbelievable."

I had found something better than beating my old time. I had found a sense of humor. I flowed up the mountain, propelled by the hilarious image of Maggie clamped onto my forearm. I focused on my breath and my center and let the energy flow through my body. It was the most relaxed and effortless uphill I had ever skied. I passed row after row of people. I tried to offer something of encouragement or humor to each person as I cruised by. It was blissful, even when my legs burned or an oxygen debt started me gasping for air again. Peach parka and black dog notwithstanding, I crossed the finish line having broken my best time by a minute. Is Time on my side or what?

Arise from sleep, old cat
And with great yawns and stretchings
Amble out of love

—Issa

Put an End to Boredom

Maybe one of the reasons that we fill up our precious time with so many activities is because we are afraid of boredom. Fear and crisis have their own formidable qualities certainly, but none as clever as boredom. Boredom is insidious, not like a mugger, a hurricane, or an angry spouse. Boredom whittles away at your desire, puts lactic acid in the muscles of your mind, devours your awareness, and drains your creativity. Boredom punctures aliveness with arrows of negative thoughts: this isn't fun, or this isn't relevant, or I'm wasting my time. Little holes maybe, but they can bleed the vitality out of their victims.

As I reflect on my childhood images of excruciating days in school watching the clock move ever so slowly, or long hot, humid summer afternoons with "nothing to do," I realize that I detested boredom. I hated feeling powerless, lacking in control.

Boredom is not the result of a certain event or situation. It is a choice you make in reaction to the situation—a choice to become

145

9

tired, disinterested, and weak. Centering is the exact opposite choice. Instead of allowing the quality of your experience to be at the mercy of a situation, you can choose a state of creativity, imagination, and adventure. Often in workshops with schools I ask teenagers to show me what boredom looks like. Within seconds they model the state exquisitely—heads lowered, major slouch, arms drooping, legs sprawled, spacey look on their faces. I test their center. There is none. They topple over and the arms go limp when I try to bend them. Then I tell them to show me what it is like when they are excited, pumped up—like getting back a test they have aced, or going into the big game and playing great. Instantly their posture is alert, their heads upright, their eyes focused and bright. I test again. They are centered and their energy is flowing. I ask them to shift between the two alternatives several times, and I point out that they can consciously choose to be bored or to be centered.

Why give up your power to a teacher, event, or life situation, simply because it is not going your way and react by creating a bored state? We know we learn quickly the things we are interested in. So always look for the connection between those things that bore us and those things we love and reframe them accordingly. Tedious housework can become a joyful, moving meditation. As we create relevancy, our energy will flow naturally. The choice always exists for you to create an energized, challenged state at any time, regardless of circumstances. No matter what humdrum may be occurring, the world you create can always be valuable and vital.

We all spend endless hours waiting—in airports, grocery lines, doctor's offices. These are ideal times to practice the art of center.

Simply sit in the waiting area quietly and breathe deeply. With each inhalation, pull energy into your being. With each exhalation, extend awareness out. Feel the body align, sit more erect, allowing gravity to flow through you, rather than on you, leaving a feeling of freedom instead of compression. Be grateful for the gift of the senses. Let the colors around you become more vivid. Study the different movement patterns of the people in the area from an

146

energetic perspective, maybe an old man shuffling along carrying the weight of history, or two little kids bubbling over with excitement and spontaneity, or harried shoppers listing lopsided under bags burgeoning with pacifiers of goodies, or teenagers loping sloppily forward with the look that only testosterone can provide. Notice if the movement is centered or uncentered.

A few more conscious breaths, and you might notice that there is a reality far beyond the various disguises of clothing and age and individual movement. There is an undercurrent, a ground of being that upholds it all. Beyond judgment flows this Ocean, its waves appearing as both the big bang of starlight and the child dancing for the pure joy of it. In that current there is no time.

Part III

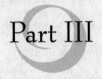

Ah, Yes!

In the vast inane there is no back or front;

The path of the bird annihilates East and West.

Day after day the sun rises in the east;

Day after day it sets in the west.

Ever onward to where the waters have an end;

Waiting motionless for when the white clouds shall arise.

Wind subsiding, the flowers still fall;

Bird crying, the mountain silence deepens.

Meeting, they laugh and laugh,

The forest grove, the many fallen leaves.

For long years a bird in a cage,

Today, flying along with the clouds.

—*Zenrin*

Slings and Arrows

*Center is knowing that everything
we need to heal is already here.*

Don't you hate colds? The trash can overflowing with crumpled tissue; all that for *one* nose? You feel like you are wearing a scuba mask. You study your schnoz in the mirror expecting to see a gigantic, swollen proboscis covering most of your face. But no, only the same old protrusion, the same one that used to be able to breathe air and smell supper.

Consider how much personal healing we've been blessed with in a lifetime. Images of fractures alone add up (well, mine do)—legs, ankles, fingers, elbows, wrists, noses, egos. And darn if they didn't all heal! Or the colds or flu, or sprains, strains, and bruises. Healed! Every one of them. And stitches and teeth knocked out—the whole growing-up-macho deal. All *healed*. You would think that we'd have developed a tremendous faith in the power of healing. But one look at the stuffed-up nose, and immediately we worry about some rare form of terminal schnozollia.

Perhaps we are too preoccupied with this dying thing. Even

in this age of unheard-of medical and technological advances, it is still true, as the rabbi said at my friend's funeral, "The ratio of life to death is still one to one." Modern society doesn't spend excessive time worrying about why we were born, so why does it always fret over the "reason" for dying? Is it this underlying fear that drives us to label every discomfort? Often labeling disease gives it power that it never deserved. Since the body is an ever-changing system, with nearly every one of its 40 trillion cells replaced yearly, who's to say that a disease isn't simply a momentary imbalance that would be corrected tomorrow if we hadn't bound it too tightly with a name and a prognosis. Is it our unconscious fear of death that keeps us so stressed in the face of life's little slings and arrows, such as health issues?

My old beliefs about health were given the acid test when my daughter, Ali, was born. By the time she was two, clothing and she no longer had a relationship. We're not talking about the typical nagging to put on a jacket because it was snowing. With her, it was a war to put on anything at all.

One winter evening Ali and I were playing cards on the living room floor. I remembered that I had to go to pick up her brother, Tommy, from ice hockey practice. The temperature was in the teens, with light snow beginning to fall. I was late and had no time for a clothing skirmish with a two-year-old. Ali, stark naked as usual, was willing to go, but *au naturel*. I looked in those stubborn two-year-old eyes, and carefully chose a light, matter-of-fact tone.

"It's cold. We have to leave to pick up Tommy. Let's put on our coats."

I put on mine and heard no complaints. I've got her now, I beamed. Wrong.

I followed her naked little buns out into the frigid air, grabbing a blanket on the way for the inevitable moment when she showed a change in attitude. I figured it would take just a few seconds.

Thank God it's dark, I thought, checking the surroundings for neighbors. As we cruised along the road, the windshield wipers swept off the falling snow, and the noisy fan blew barely enough heat to defrost the windshield.

"There's a blanket on the back seat if you need it," I reminded her in my most nonchalant tone.

"Ali's a good girl," she replied, speaking about herself in the third person, a habit perfected by two-year-olds.

And then she started singing a song from *Sesame Street,* "C is for Cookie, that's good enough for me."

I began to wonder if singing had been genetically developed by our cave-dwelling ancestors to endure life's harsh elements. I glanced at Ali. Maybe my little songster was a reincarnated samurai growing strong through voluntary hard training. The ancient samurai knew the importance of embracing death so that he could fully embrace life. (Of course, the average life span back then was twenty-nine years.) Or maybe she was just a stubborn pre-schooler with a pushover daddy. All I knew for certain was that at that moment my hands were freezing and thank goodness I didn't see any cops.

When we drove up in front of the rink, Tommy jumped into the seat next to Ali.

"Ali!" he laughed. "Did you forget something?"

He scrutinized both of us, recognizing immediately by our resolute expressions that a strange truce was in place. He wrapped his arm around his naked sister.

Her eyes showed fierce determination: "Ali's not cold." (And why is it that two-year-olds talk in the third person?)

Her communication was clear. She was a big girl and could make decisions for herself.

Slump-shouldered, I followed her bare feet into the house, dragging my blanket behind me. And days later I watched for signs of pneumonia. Not even a sniffle.

Our beliefs are fundamental to the healing process. Coming

153

from a traditional upbringing, I had my share: "Stay in bed"; "Listen to your doctor"; "Take the prescribed medication." I assumed they were true. So my "healing" beliefs were firmly entrenched by the time I was a teenager. Then I met Cathy.

Cathy was seventeen when we were introduced. She possessed more energy, spirit, and vitality than anybody I had ever seen. She seemed to take more physical risks than even my buddies, who were definitely on the edge. She jumped out of trees, tripped down stairs, did flips off of cliffs into quarries (usually water-filled) for fun, and generally hung out with me, which was dangerous in itself, without ever an injury or sick day. Oh, she must have had bruises or strains here, a cold or headache there. But she didn't know it. By that, I mean, she didn't let it interfere with her life, gave it no energy. Over the years I never saw her take any medicine or even go to a doctor. Asking her about this led me to her grandmother.

Cathy's grandmother was a Christian healer who believed that all sickness could be healed through prayer and good thought. The world looked on these people as fanatics, as in the old joke about the guy caught in a flood on the roof of his home. When a man in a rowboat came by to rescue him, he refused the offer, saying that God would save him. Hours later, with water continuing to rise, he denied a motorboat attempt, saying "God will save me." With water up to his neck and hanging on to the chimney, a helicopter flew over for one last attempt. "God will save me," he shouted, waving the chopper away.

He drowned. Upon arriving at the pearly gates he was rather angry.

"St. Peter," he demanded, "why didn't God save me?"

St. Peter shook his head sadly. "What do you mean? He sent you two boats and a helicopter."

Having limped and sneezed my way through life, I wanted to meet this grandmother. One Christmas, I had my chance. In her seventies, "G.G," as she was affectionately known by her relatives, was no small woman. Cooking and eating, in that order, were her hobbies. Dining at her place was a feast even at snack time. I liked her immediately. Her love and compassion and pound cake made a permanent impact on me. As a kid, I had been in deep states of reverence and connection often— dreaming in my tree house, running barefoot through the grass, going untouched in tag football, lying (briefly) on the bottom of the pool pretending to be a fish. Deeply centered states. G.G. understood these as "spiritual" states. To Cathy and the other family members, she was just grandmother, with those funny habits and eccentricities that go with grandfolks everywhere. But she was new spiritual territory for me, and I wanted to know what she had that made her "different."

For one thing, she slept very little, staying up late at night praying for healing for her many patients across the country. From time to time, I would call her and, in more than one instance, experience an immediate healing for ailments that ranged from severe pain to depression. The instantaneous change in my health challenged my belief that healing takes time. According to G.G., the imbalances of life that we call sickness or injury are simply products of wrong thinking, of addictions to the physical world. But when we correct our thinking, sickness loses its power in the face of "divine intelligence." This is not just Christian-based thinking. The Hindus might call this illusory physical world "maya," or merely a smoke screen hiding the reality of the "absolute, unbounded ocean of God."

In spite of her strong beliefs, G.G. wasn't a fanatic. During college I injured my knee playing football. The doctors diagnosed severe cartilage and ligament damage and declared that an operation was imperative. When I consulted Grandmother, she suggested "that all things can be healed, if the faith and belief are there. But we must also use common sense in applying these principles." She recommended that I go ahead and have the operation. There was no imparting of guilt or sense of failure. Just love, the essence of all her teachings.

Even my daughter, Ali, seemed to understand the principle of mind over matter. When she was ten, she was a dedicated gymnast. She had an opportunity to qualify in Denver for a regional meet in Arkansas. The afternoon before, she was practicing for a school-wide talent show and landed incorrectly on her ankle, twisting it. She had continued the routine as if nothing was wrong. When I saw her backstage, she was limping painfully. The ankle was swollen and tender to the touch. I applied ice.

"Ali, you've got to listen to your body. If it's an injury, maybe it would be best to rest it."

One look at that determined little face, and I knew that there was no doubt in her mind about doing the performance that evening.

"We at least need to tape it," I conceded. "It'll give you added support."

By evening she could barely walk, hobbling about on her toes. I taped her ankle, consciously holding back a very strong tendency to make another arbitrary parental ruling. I had witnessed too many unexplainable healings to deny anyone with conviction, especially my daughter, the opportunity to go for it. My only suggestion was to get centered, breathe, and extend energy.

"Okay, Dad. I'll be fine. Don't worry."

Heck, somebody's got to worry, right?

Ali went through the performance beautifully, with only a few minor adjustments and some wobbles on landing a back layout. It was difficult for me to imagine how anyone could perform leaps and flips with such a painful injury. Immediately following the performance, she was limping badly. Surely she would have to call off going to Denver for the gymnastic qualifying meet. Wrong again.

"Dad, don't worry!"

I began to consider that this whole thing could be some kind of an act, to make her performance seem more incredible than it was. As a schoolteacher, I had seen many young children her age fake injuries for the strokes and sympathy. But she had rarely exhibited that drama, except when she was much younger and had an addiction for multicolored Band-Aids. And besides, I had seen a lot of ankles in my day, and this one was not a pretty sight. I sat on a chair backstage, holding her ankle and applying kiatsu, a healing technique that I had learned from Koichi Tohei Sensei. But within minutes she was up, giving me a quick hug, and hobbling off with her gymnastic friends to an awaiting van for the four-hour drive to Denver.

Two days later she returned. She had managed to qualify for the regionals! She was beaming. And limping just like when she had left.

"Great job. But tomorrow, young lady [big trouble when I use that phrase], we're going to get an X-ray."

The next day the verdict was in. Broken ankle.

"There's no way she'll be doing anything with that ankle for several weeks," the doctor said.

"How about backflips?" I said with a wink to Ali.

Centering had helped Ali deal with injury while not curtailing her performance. But, in her case, it wasn't the conscious physical centering that was so effective, even though she said she used it. It was her centered purpose that did the trick. Her intent to do both the talent show and regional gymnastic meet far outweighed the discomfort in her ankle. Her centered vision was much stronger than her temporary affliction, and her congruent mind-body state protected her and gave her the vitality she needed.

In a slightly more famous event in 1996, Kerri Strug overcame a serious sprain and applied that same thinking in landing a vault to help win the gold medal for the U.S. Olympic Team.

ⵔ ⵔ ⵔ

Other than my Mom's major bout with polio when I was five, I can't remember my parents ever being too ill to get out of bed. During all those years of growing up I can only recall one time when my Dad was in bed past 6:30 A.M., and all he had was a twenty-four-hour flu. They were up with the sun every morning, a habit I ardently avoided as a youth. Meanwhile, my folks are in their eighties and nineties now. I still haven't caught them sick in bed.

Except for once.

I was in San Diego, California, doing a two-day public workshop. At the end of the first day I gathered the participants in a circle for a closing meditation. As we sat in silence, I noticed that my foot was swelling and becoming quite sore. Although my eyes remained closed, I could feel the familiar throb of a serious sprain or break. It must be in my imagination, I concluded, knowing that I had not felt any pain prior to sitting down and couldn't recall injuring myself at all during the last several days. "It must be just a cramp or swollen feet, like after a long plane flight," I concluded. I wiggled my foot and rolled my ankle around. Ouch! It could hardly roll and certainly ached. After ringing the bell at the end of the twenty-minute sitting period, I opened my eyes. To my amazement the left ankle was much larger than the right.

I said my good-byes from my chair. After the people had departed, I looked at my assistant, Ellen Stapenhorst, and the coordinator of the event, Robin Blanc.

"I don't think I can walk. Look at the size of this ankle!"

"When did that happen?" Robin exclaimed.

"While I was meditating," I laughed, hoping that my levity might make it disappear.

"Oh, come on," urged Ellen. "Did you land funny in that last demo?"

"Not to my knowledge," I said. I too wondered what I did. Previous injuries of this nature had happened during a distinct moment, like getting blindsided by an opposing linebacker. But there had been none this time. And, more important, could I walk, and how was I going to continue this workshop, full of movement and aikido, the next day? Using Ellen and Robin for support, I hobbled to the car. We drove to a dinner party that Robin had planned in my honor.

Doing the kind of work that I do, I am accustomed to having many friends whose profession is healing—physicians, chiropractors, acupuncturists, herbalists, therapists, you name it. Being in Southern California increased the number manyfold. Before I knew it, I was lying in the middle of Robin's living room, besieged by a dozen people, each with a surefire cure for my ailment. Within a three-hour period I had ice packs, herbal wraps, acupuncture needles, cranial adjustments, homeopathic drops under my tongue, laying on of hands, prayers, crystals spinning above my ankle, colored-light therapy, and some strange healing sounds to create "harmonic resonance." I accepted them all with gratitude, if not guilt.

"Every remedy and religion has been represented here. If I don't heal by tomorrow, I'm a real schmuck!"

The next morning I swung my feet over the side of the bed to see the miracle healing. Alas, still swollen. I took one gingerly painful step before grabbing the bedpost. I considered my dilemma. The lesson must not be to demonstrate miraculous healing, but instead to show that sprained ankles don't stop a seminar, even if it's on movement and peak performance. I needed to get centered, breathe deeply, let go of my embarrassment, and focus on adding value! Not easy when you have images of people booing and walking out on this charlatan pretending to teach mind-body coordination. I hobbled on stage with crutches and a twisted smile.

Even from my chair, the session flowed. Ellen did the physical demonstrations beautifully. The audience was wonderfully supportive. The work was getting done even without me doing it. More important than a good leg were good friends.

At the end of the day Robin dropped me off at the airport. My ankle was markedly better. I didn't need the crutches. Even more miraculous, the next morning when I awoke in Colorado, I had no swelling or soreness. My ankle was fine, not just for walking, but for aikido, skiing, anything. In my whole life I had never experienced such unwarranted incapacitation followed by such rapid healing.

One week later I got a call from Mom and Dad. Dad's voice was not as strong and vital as usual. After a few minutes of general chitchat I mentioned it.

"You sound different, Dad. Are you all right?"

"Well, I had a little accident a week ago. I was in the hospital."

"Yeah, in critical condition!" piped in Mom, wanting to get the whole truth out.

"What! You've got to be kidding!" I shouted. "How come you didn't call me sooner?"

"I call you when I feel good, not when I feel lousy," replied Dad. "Besides, I'm fine now. Knew I would be."

"What happened?"

There was a pause.

"My golfing partner ran me over with the golf cart."

I burst out laughing with the image, relieved that they sounded so at ease.

"Yeah, the cart didn't just run him over. It smashed him into the clubhouse wall."

"Dad," I chuckled, "you must have beat him pretty bad."

"Nah, he didn't mean to do it. But you know how we old farts are. I was just leaning down to tie my golf shoes, and Mel goes to back up the cart. Only he puts it in forward, not reverse. Next thing I know I wake up in the critical care unit with tubes sticking out of me."

160

"Well, what did happen to you?"

"A ringing head, some good bruises, a bunch of cracked ribs, and worst of all, a severely broken ankle."

"A broken ankle?" I shouted. "Which one?"

"Left."

That explained it.

"What the heck does it matter right or left?"

I told him the story of my ankle. They were amazed. I was dumbfounded.

"Dad, I know you don't want to call me when you are feeling lousy. But you've got to. It'll save me a lot of pain."

The event left me awake at night. There was no way that the cells of my ankle were in instantaneous communication with my father's. Was there? But I had read about the work of Dr. David Bohm, a physicist noted for his research in quantum mechanics. According to physicists, in the subatomic world, the distinction between matter and energy dissolves. Particles of matter often behave like waves, and waves of energy may behave like particles. Inside the atom these wave-particle packages, called quanta, act like little magicians. Quanta can jump from one orbit of an atom to another orbit, without passing through the space in between. It is, as science writer John Briggs states, "like a rabbit appearing and disappearing in two different hats." Furthermore, "when researchers would fire a stream of particles at a screen with two slits in it, each particle seemed to be able to go through two slits at the same time. When paired particles were separated in space, they were somehow able to communicate instantaneously with each other, like the Corsican Brothers—the Siamese twins who, though separated at birth, retained a connection so direct that when one was slashed by a sword, the other in a faraway city felt the pain."

At the quantum level, healing prayer work and the ankle-to-ankle communication with my father might be understandable. How would our overall state of health change if we could integrate the quantum principles into our daily life? One thing is for certain—the cellular phone business would be in big trouble.

> *Consider the lilies how they grow; they toil not, they spin not; and yet I say that Solomon in all his glory was not arrayed like one of these. If then God so clothe the grass, which is today in the field, and tomorrow is cast in the oven; how much more will he clothe you, O ye of little faith?"*
>
> —Matthew 6:28–30

THINK HEALTHY

Great health is not simply the absence of disease. It's having abundant energy and freedom to fulfill your potential. For this reason great health can't be separated into compartments. It is an expression of the unity of mind, body, and spirit. And what may be lacking in one area can be brought back into dynamic balance by the others—just watch a runner in the Special Olympics exuberantly crossing the finish line.

We are finally beginning to break through to new paradigms of health and healing. Thanks to physician- and healer-authors such as Andrew Weil, Larry Dossey, Deepak Chopra, Norman Cousins, Bernie Siegel, O. Carl Simonton, among many others, we are learning that seeing ourselves and believing ourselves to be whole, healthy, balanced, and vital has a medical and scientific basis in creating optimum health.

Oak Ridge Laboratories concluded through radioisotope studies that you replace 98 percent of the total number of your atoms every year. Every cell in the body is replaced over time. You have a new stomach lining every five days, you have a new skin cover every five weeks, and the "solid" skeleton is recycled every three months. Even the physical director of the show, the cell's DNA—that tiny, twisting double-helix strand that resides in every one of the 40

trillion cells in your body—is not spared. So what's left? According to Deepak Chopra, M.D., the only aspect that is retained in this
ever-changing human entity is intelligence, or memory. It's not
physical stuff. It is nonstuff or "consciousness" that makes sure that
a skin cell becomes a skin cell, a heart cell becomes a heart cell,
and a tree continues as a tree.

I personally find it comforting to know that who I really am is
nonstuff.

Dr. Chopra says that if you were diagnosed with liver cancer you
should know that every cell of the liver will renew within six weeks.
And, when you consider how many times that healthy liver cell had
reproduced itself over your life as compared to the replication of
the abnormal or diseased cell, the possibility of changing the memory or intelligence of a liver cell back to its powerful healthy state
is quite real indeed. Therefore, your conscious thoughts and beliefs
have a direct effect on your cell's memory, or intelligence, and
therefore your health. It is the one consistent key that runs through
all the healthy people that I've been associated with—they "think
healthy."

Entertain positive thoughts regarding your health and change
any negative ones quickly when they appear. For example, "You'll
catch your death of cold" or "I'm worried sick over . . ." are probably
not the best programming you can give your subconscious, or your
children for that matter. If you have to be in nasty weather, then
think of the cold or wet as invigorating, actually stimulating and
strengthening the immune system. Take faith from the children in
any community who, whenever it's a cold miserable morning, are
still in sneakers, T-shirts, and *maybe* a jacket—unzipped of course.
And they are just as healthy as the superinsulated kids whose Moms
prepared them for a Himalayan expedition when they're just going
to the school bus. Kids can get those coughs that sound like a frog
over the PA system, the kind of cough that will keep us worried
adults honking away for weeks. And, despite playing all day in
nasty weather, kids can still emerge from their bedroom the next

morning vibrantly healthy and cough-free. What's the message here? It's that beliefs play a much larger role in our health than degrees Fahrenheit. (And, I still wear a coat and hat when it's cold and nasty. Personally, I *like* to stay warm and dry.)

Healthy food is important, but a healthy attitude is more so. You will receive the maximum benefit inherent in any food if you center, eat with awareness, appreciating what you have, and being thankful for those who are providing it.

One morning while visiting my folks, I hobbled into the kitchen stiff from my aerobics, aching from yesterday's weight training, eyes bagged over from last night's emotional releasing, looking for my ovo-free spirulina and lactose-free soy milk to wash down my truckload of whole-food supplement pills.

"Do you want a sweet roll to go with your eggs?"

"No thanks, Mom."

"What? You don't like eggs?" barked Dad.

"They'll put some meat on those bones," chirped Mom.

"What the heck is wrong with eggs?" Dad was relentless. "Never bothered me."

I rummaged through a shelf looking for the oat bran. I knew there was no way out of this predicament. How could I possibly give a lecture on proper nutrition to my Dad, or my Mom for that matter? I turned my whole body around to look at my folks. (I would have just turned my neck but it was too stiff.) Eighty-five and ninety years old, awake hours before me, lean, mean, supersenior machines. Pictures of health, they eat three square meals a day, never missing a dessert. Eight A.M., noon, and six. You can set your clock by it. In these modern eggless, dairyless, meatless days, they could care less. They eat everything and like it. So who was I kidding?

I looked at my Mom's happy face and put the oat bran back on the shelf. It would still be there tomorrow.

"Okay, Mom. Gimme a sweet roll. And a plate of eggs. Scrambled."

The most powerful, healthy thoughts come when you take the time to center, to sit quietly and dive down into that ocean of consciousness that flows through, and is the source of, all of life. It is this deep ocean of universal intelligence that can manifest thoughts and intentions instantaneously. It is at this level that the mind, body, and spirit unify. For instance, when you cut yourself, the mind and body automatically coagulate the blood and form new skin tissue.

Just imagine if you had to rely on surface thinking to do the job. "Boss, I can't come to work this month, I'm busy grafting ten million new skin cells for this blister I broke open."

In science we have learned that if you lower the temperature of something close to absolute zero, it becomes superconductive, meaning that the electrons flow unrestricted, indefinitely. There is no resistance. Similarly, as your mind settles down to deeper levels of calmness, the natural harmony of mind, body, and spirit happens effortlessly. Life force flows wherever it is needed.

Within both intergalactic space and your own mind-body lurks a power that can create a sun, form a galaxy, or completely transform any aspect of physical and mental experience. To tap into this superintelligence is the next great adventure for humankind.

Centered Relationship

We are the boat
We are the sea
I sail in you
You sail in me.

—*Pete Seeger*

I don't usually eavesdrop. But not long ago at a restaurant in the Toronto airport, I pretended not to notice the couple sitting at the table next to mine. The man had asked the woman a question, using a sharp voice, the kind of voice which implies that, no matter what her answer, she was wrong.

"Yes," had been her retort, cold and lifeless, taunting him with obvious disinterest as she toyed deliberately with the baked potato on her plate.

Those were the first words I had heard them speak in the twenty minutes that they had been there. In their forties, they appeared invisible to one another. It was as if they were eating alone, occasionally looking at the comings and goings of others, or staring blankly into their food, resigned and resentful.

I too was eating alone, but enjoying it immensely. I think that either one of them would have gladly changed places with me, trading loneliness for aloneness.

With a cup of hot soup, and pen and notepad in hand—and a four-hour layover—I was perched in an ideal crow's nest for observing people. My intention to edit a chapter in this book was upstaged by my fascination with this unhappy couple, and also with two other couples who had entered the restaurant.

The couple seated on my left were young and attractive, consumed by their romance. Anything said by one was met with enthusiasm and a smile by the other. They were at the top of their charm games, touching and flirting, the water fountain flowing behind me a mere trickle compared to their raging hormones. And now *I* was beginning to feel lonely, and a part of me wanted to trade places with them. I glanced again at the first couple, those silent human statues on my right, and for a moment I erased twenty years from their faces and imagined them happily together in a romance dance of their own. What had happened to change all of that?

And then, directly in front of me by the window sat a third couple—a couple probably in their mid-sixties. They also were relatively quiet, but they seemed content and together in their silence. They weren't seated facing one another, but next to each other around one corner of the table. They spoke softly, listened sincerely. Occasionally, they touched—a hand on a hand or a hand on a shoulder. They weren't overflowing with excitement and animation like the young lovers, but neither were they so self-absorbed. They just appeared to be enjoying each other.

Their sense of connection ran deep and contained a certain selflessness. They weren't so consumed that they couldn't give full attention to the waiter and would periodically point to things outside the window. My reaction to this couple was one of respect, sensing the depth and wisdom in their relationship.

I am quite certain that none of the couples realized that I was chronicling their Toronto restaurant behavior. Nor were they aware that they had given me a gift—information for writing

167

about centered relationship. More than just observing the couples, I saw myself in each one of them. Haven't you also been there?

At the root of centered relationship are two people who are able to be centered with or without the other. The exchange of energy, whether it is an idea, a feeling, or an action, flows from an aligned state of mind, body, and spirit, unhindered by neediness. When we are centered as individuals, we are able to unconditionally accept and love who we are and have a natural commitment to personal growth. Only then are we prepared to enter relationship in a similar loving and supportive way, devoid of controlling and manipulative behaviors.

Centering is a lifelong process for each of us. Likewise, centered relationship takes time and daily practice. It is the most rigorous growth training of all. And the most fulfilling. And yet it is easy to get consumed by a sound bite, quick-fix world that does not encourage us to mindfully explore relationship. If the romantic couple in the restaurant is unable to see that relationship is a growing and changing process, they are likely to run to the exit door at the first sign of struggle, long before the opportunity to experience the type of joy that the oldest couple was getting.

In the romantic phase we often confuse falling in love and loving.

When we fall in love, we do feel an ecstatic feeling, don't we? We feel a wonderful quality of connectedness, an extraordinary moment, moment after moment.

But what happens when we "fall" in love is that we believe that the extraordinary moment is caused by something outside of ourselves, by a particular person or situation. We begin to think that the power of that loving experience is caused by the "form"—the person or situation—so we feel compelled to replicate it. As Stewart Emery says in *Actualizations: You Don't Have to Rehearse to Be Yourself:* When we say 'I'm falling in love with you,' we are really saying 'I am becoming the effect of you, and it's more fun than being the effect of the dreary stuff I am usually the effect of.'"As we go through life attached to specific forms that we think enable us to experience love, the lock on our hearts becomes ever more complicated. Many friends my age have confessed that they are now "too set in their ways" and have too many conditions to ever find a relationship that works. The key to a heart like this becomes more and more complex over time, and before too long, only the most perfect person can open it. And that person, it seems, is always already taken!

The real key is to work on ourselves. When we are centered, we recognize that what is really happening when we fall in love is that the form—the person, the event—just happened to touch the place inside us that is love. The awareness that the essence of relationship is inside of us brings us to center and allows us to appreciate the form without clinging to it.

Without awareness and honest exploration, we continue to struggle with the form, creating relationships that are full of conditions, molded in the mud of societal pressure and personal neediness: I need or expect you to behave in a certain manner, play a certain role (husband/wife, mother/father, housekeeper/breadwinner), look a certain way, and, by the way, "Don't ever change."

Huh? No wonder most relationships dissolve. Nationally, fifty-five out of every hundred marriages end in divorce. We feel betrayed when our expectations aren't met. Power struggles ensue to force each person back into the "picture" of how he or she is viewed by the other. Could this have been the struggle that was shutting down couple number one? The endless battle over which person is "right" reminded me of Archie Bunker's marital wisdom: "The only thing that holds a marriage together is the husband being big enough to step back and see where the wife was wrong."

These power struggles should fail. Relationships based on conditions derived from neediness and dependency aren't fulfilling. They don't support growth. They aren't nurturing. They aren't centered.

And yet, it only takes one person who has the courage to be centered to begin a centered relationship. There once was a very wise monk who lived in the sixteenth century in Japan whose name was Stichiri. He was sitting one day in meditation in his austere little home when a thief broke in. The monk was so quiet that the thief didn't even realize that he was there. As the thief was busy sneaking around the room, looting, he suddenly heard a sound.

"Excuse me, sir, but could you be a little quieter? I am meditating here."

Thoroughly unnerved at this, the thief drew a sword, "I am going to cut your head off if you make a move."

The monk raised his hand calmly and said, "Please, take whatever you like, don't be afraid, just be a little more quiet, I am meditating."

Then he went right back into his meditation.

Totally off-centered by this, the thief looted his way with one eye warily cast on this strange monk. Just as he was ready to open the door to leave, he heard, "Excuse me. But I do have some rent to pay this week. Could you please leave a little for that. Thank you."

Disarmed, the thief reached into his own pocket and pulled out some money. Just as he was about to go out the door, the monk spoke: "Don't you think that when someone gives you something, you should thank him for it?"

Nervously, the thief mumbled, "Thank you," slammed the door, and ran.

170

The thief was caught a couple of weeks later robbing another house. When he was brought to trial, the monk was asked to testify. The judge told the monk, "Please explain how this man robbed you."

The monk looked up at the judge and at the man lovingly,

"This man didn't rob me, I gave him everything, and he thanked me for it."

With that the monk left the courtroom.

The thief was convicted, however, because of other testimony and spent two years in prison. The day he was released, he went directly to the monk and became one of his most devoted disciples.

The monk, Tsuchiri, *chose* centered relationship. He wasn't hoping or searching for a centered relationship. He *was* centered relationship. It started with his relationship to himself and naturally expanded to the universe around him.

We begin to realize that we can consciously choose to make that centered, loving place inside much bigger, so that no matter where we go, whether we turn here and see a flower, turn there and see a child, here and see an "enemy," all forms touch the place in us that is love. That place becomes so big that we can't help but become constantly anchored in loving relationship, centered relationship. We don't have to "own" the form, or control and manipulate the situation in any way. Everything about the form is a gift, an opportunity for us to learn and to serve compassionately.

There was a very revered monk named Takuan, who lived in feudal Japan upon a mountain overlooking a fishing village. One day he noticed a group of angry villagers outside his poor little hut. He emerged smiling, "Good day, my friends."

And they looked at him with disgust. The leader of the village spoke.

"How can one monk who is so revered do such a despicable act? A thirteen-year-old girl has just recently had a child and she admitted that the father of the child is you. How could you do such a sinful thing when you preach the exact opposite? It is your responsibility to take care of this child."

The monk looked at them, his heart full of compassion, and said, "Is that so?"

He held his hands out to receive the child, and carried the infant back into his hut.

Now the monk was a very poor man, but he gave the child great love. He did everything in his power to feed and clothe the child. He nurtured and cared for that young child with every ounce of his being. The child blossomed.

After about a year the monk looked out from his hut and once more saw the villagers gathered outside. But this time they were on their knees bowing. The monk, with the little child in his arms, emerged smiling,

"Good day, my friends!"

The leader looked up, "Please forgive us, Master. We have greatly wronged you. The young girl has admitted that she lied to us, and that the true father was a young fisherman from a nearby village. They have decided to marry and have asked for their child back."

The monk, his heart full of compassion, said, "Is that so?"

He handed them the child, bowed with deep love, and returned to his hut.

Given our modern life, the behavior of the two monks can be difficult to comprehend. And yet there are opportunities every day to explore these same teachings in simple ways.

I remember when my son, Tommy, wanted to leave home after the ninth grade and go away to school in Minnesota to play ice hockey. My personal desire to not lose him to the world so quickly was strong, and I could have attempted to influence him or demand that he stay. I needed to get centered to see that my personal neediness did not interfere with the greater responsibility of supporting his growth.

My first concern was that this was something Tommy really wanted to do. His reply was consistent:

"I'll miss you guys. But I love hockey and it'll give me the best opportunity to find out how good I can be." Each time we would discuss it, he would be more centered and congruent about his desire. My choice was made much easier.

"Well, then, I'll support you in whatever way you need to make that happen. What do we need to do?"

The initiative and responsibility to make it happen were his. He selected a prep school with a fine hockey program in Minneapolis, and wrote the headmaster and a major sponsor of the school's hockey program.

There was no reply for weeks. I began to lose my center, discouraged by the thought that they disregarded the handwritten letter, considering it too unprofessional, and that they had dashed Tommy's courageous thoughts to step forward in life. But Tommy seemed to have no fears about the delay. And then one evening a man called to say he was a supporter of the hockey program and had received a powerful letter from a young man and could he talk to him. He was in Aspen and would like to come to one of Tommy's games.

On a tearful day the following September I said good-bye to Tommy as he boarded a plane to Minneapolis. Three years later he was back in Colorado playing Division I hockey with Colorado College.

In relationship, whether it is man-woman, parent-child, or among friends, we are there to set the other free, and not impose upon them any more chains than they are already wearing. This is not an easy thing to do. In fact, it's one of the hardest.

When we are uncentered in relationship, we must have the courage to ask for support. When Tommy was eighteen, I felt that, as a parent, I was tentative and insecure when I was around him. There was some tension, a certain lack of comfort when we were in the same room. I felt judgment—I of him and he of me. When I took the time to center and to look inside—at me and not at him—I realized that my discomfort came from lack of confidence that I felt in my parenting. I wasn't sure where the

173

balance point was between letting him be his own man and providing some structure. It became clear that I needed some support from Tommy in freeing me of any unnecessary chains that I was imposing upon myself.

I began to look for the right moment to discuss this delicate subject. This is not always easy. We are used to seeing conflict as a contest or as something negative. As a result we don't bring it up until those times in which we are so upset or angry that we can't deny it anymore. And in that tense, contracted state we are assured of inappropriate communication that only deepens the problem.

One evening I felt that we were both in a centered state, relaxing on the porch after dinner. This is how I remember our conversation.

"Tommy," I asked, "is this a good time to discuss something that I need your help with?"

"Yeah, sure," said Tommy, looking directly at me for the first time since sitting down, and curious, since fathers are more famous for giving lectures rather than asking for help.

"Well, then, here's my dilemma. When we're together, I feel like I've been walking around on eggshells. You're just out of high school, and I've never been the dad of an eighteen-year-old before. I'm not sure how to be a father in this new role. When you're out partying or doing something that I think may be unhealthy or unwise, like some of the things I did at eighteen, for example, I'm not sure how to tell you in a way that honors your age and need for independence and my role as Dad. I'm walking a tightrope between providing freedom and providing structure."

"Yeah?" said Tommy in a way that sounded like "What the heck are you talking about?" It's poignant how quickly a teenager can puncture a well-rehearsed plan for deep bonding.

But I was committed.

"So, I'm asking for your support. Would you coach me? I want you to give me feedback about what's working and what isn't. And I really need permission to make mistakes, to overlecture sometimes or be undiplomatic about how I say things, which could happen when I'm worried about your welfare. And I need you to tell me your experience of whether I'm on target or out of line. I want to be the best possible Dad. I know you want to be the best possible son. If we can tell our truth without the unnecessary judging of each other, if we can learn to be tough on the issue, but soft on the person, I think we could even learn to appreciate our differences, and have more fun in the process."

"Okay, Dad, I hear you." He paused, "And, by the way, I think you're doing pretty great." No heavy coaching tips, no deep bonding, no tears. Just some awkward silence.

And then he said, "I've got to go over to Coley's now. Is that all right?"

"Sure. And thanks," I said as he hopped off the steps and bounded into the car, shouting, "You bet!"

What happened? Nothing special on the surface. We didn't walk off together holding hands in a field of flowers. We didn't start spending more time together in late-night philosophical discussions. In fact, I recently asked Tommy about this very poignant moment in my parenting life. His reply was "Yeah, I sort of remember the conversation." But on the other hand, I never again had the feeling of walking on eggshells.

Appreciation of differences is an essential part of centered relationship. For instance, writing a book does not come easily for me. One of the problems is that my life partner, Cathy, is a good critical reader. You would think that she and I would make a pretty good team when it comes to writing a book. But if "pretty good" means a smooth and harmonious literary relationship, forget it. At some point, starting with my first book, and continuing through most of this one, Cathy developed a severe distaste for reading my proofs. By her own admission she would show irritation, even anger, at the prospect of having to edit my

175

9

work. It did wonders for my self-esteem as a writer. Yet Cathy's criticism was simply too valuable to pass up. If I didn't have the tools to make this aspect of my relationship work, of what value would be this chapter?

Cathy's one of those people who reads the *New Yorker* from cover to cover each week, marvels while reading the great writers like Steinbeck and D. H. Lawrence, gags at the thought of airplane novels, and wants to burn all how-to books. Obviously, the perfect quality control person for me. And my worst editing nightmare. Even as I'm writing this, I see old images of bold red markings: "What's your point?"; "Huh?"; "Rewrite!"; or a large red X across an entire page. She is ruthless.

I can handle all this most of the time, figuring that if she liked it, it must be good. But if she didn't like something that I was convinced was good, I couldn't just subtly leave it in. I needed and wanted her approval—a fact that was actually a big acknowledgment of her. But what would happen was that we'd go to battle. And she would often experience that as my unwillingness to listen to and acknowledge her thoughts, and she would simply refuse to edit anymore. I was left staring at a chapter with a bunch of red marks, and an uncentered relationship.

One day after meditating I was sitting on the floor with a pile of papers of old drafts. The history of red "Fix this!" or "Oh, please!" or "You can do better than this" painted a hilarious picture of our predicament. Our perspectives were too limited around who got to be right. The humor of it all suddenly dawned, and a way out of the problem seemed clear. I began to point out TV ads, movies, or magazine articles that were poorly written, and I would stamp them with one of Cathy's famous red-mark quotes. Over time the "Oh, please" and "What's the point?" became funny, and we started laughing together at our dilemma. I gave up needing to prove my point, and she felt acknowledged for her valuable input.

One day, as I was editing this chapter, this note dropped out of the last draft, which, not ironically, turned out to be the last chapter written:

Dear Tommy,

There was a period of time when I was sure we would not be able to do this project—edit your book—together. But now that it is essentially complete, I have to tell you something.

You were the one who made it work out. You were the one who was able to get centered about it and break the negative pattern we were stuck in. When I got angry and vented my anger by rolling my eyes, and groaning out loud and saying, "Oh, please," when I thought a passage was trite, you somehow found a way to laugh.

I'm really glad you were able to do this, because I had no idea how much I wanted to be part of your book. Now, even though I still groan now and then, I like what it teaches.

Love, Cathy

I resisted putting this letter in the book because it sounded like I was tooting my horn, but my esteemed resident editor disagreed.

> If there were just one gift I could give to you,
> I would stand as a mirror to your life,
> and you would see the way you've grown,
> see the way you shine,
> and see all the love that's in your eyes.

—*Ellen Stapenhorst*

CREATE CENTERED RELATIONSHIPS

Have you ever looked at a person, even someone you may see every-day, and yet at that moment experienced him or her as extraordinary, even divine? And you may wonder why at other times you missed seeing this quality.

When you give something your conscious attention, when you bring You to It, something changes. Centered relationship does not depend on a particular person. It is a quality of being that you bring to that person. You are choosing to appreciate another from center.

The more centered you are, the more aware you are. The more aware, the more deeply you connect to another. The more deeply you connect, the more you appreciate another. The more you appreciate, the more joyful you become. The more joyful you become, the more willing to deepen that relationship. And the cycle begins anew, with more depth.

When you are centered, you recognize that the relationship you have with another is bigger and grander than the garbage often generated by your differences, and that taking out the garbage is a worthwhile practice. It is one of the best opportunities we have for personal growth and for strengthening the relationship. The first questions you should ask yourself when the garbage of conflict appears are, "Am I centered? Am I coming from a place of love or fear, being open or being right?"

Then, from this more compassionate place, ask, "What do I need to learn?"

These questions will help you gain perspective and wisdom in the face of conflict, and will be reflected in a more centered choice of words and deeds, further strengthening the relationship.

For example, if someone releases a barrage of unreasonable demands, it is important not to choose a reactive state of defensiveness and retaliation. Breathe deeply from center and sincerely listen, aware of not just the words, but also the feelings, the physiology, and any hidden message. Make careful mental notes of the specific demands the person is making, and if you have their permission, even take written notes. When he or she is finished, ask if you could recap the main points to see if you heard it all correctly. If this is done in an authentic and compassionate way, you may be surprised when the individual takes the initiative to change the unreasonable demands to more appropriate requests. The person often will clean up his language and harshness and even apologize. A recentering will be established without force if you will give up resisting attackers and help them to see precisely where their negative energy is taking them.

Don't expect centered relationship to always look like you want it to. In the story of my son Tommy when he was eighteen, you might have wondered whether he stopped staying out late? No. But I learned that wasn't the problem, just like a messy room or a poor grade in school isn't the problem. When I looked inside, I recognized that the fundamental problem was my concern over being the best possible parent, one who nurtures responsible, resourceful, and respectful human beings. If I could look into a crystal ball, and see that when my kids are adults they will be responsible, happy people, then certain teenage habits wouldn't bother me so much.

Deep down inside, every person wants to be responsible, resourceful, and respectful. They just might have different criteria about what that looks like, and a clean room might not be one of them. Honest and centered communication allows us to recognize our different criteria and support each other in the common goal of becoming happy and caring human beings.

This means that a true centered relationship has no permanent conditions, rules, expectations, or criteria as its basis. You are in relationship with another for the magnificent opportunity of discovering and creating who you really are (the highest and happiest concept of yourself), and for enjoying and supporting the other's discovery and creation of who he or she is.

If the creations begin to conflict, then there is the grand opportunity and challenge to gather up your courage and choose to be centered enough to honor and not judge the other for what he has created and what paths he is choosing. It may even necessitate changing the form of the relationship, that is, dissolving a traditional marriage relationship or living together situation for something entirely different in order to support that path. And if done in a loving, honest manner, the result can be a relationship that will grow even stronger. Because there were no conditions or expectations that hindered each person's ability to live his or her highest truth, the two see in each other a true, loving friend who in truth is always there. This is centered relationship.

When you find yourself in pain, or even in intense dislike in a relationship, it's easy to stay shut down and be right, even righteous. It takes strong courage in those moments to reach over and touch that person lovingly. Get centered and do it anyway, knowing that somewhere behind that cloud of anger is a boundless sky of love.

Almost Gone
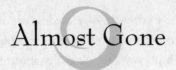

He not busy being born
is busy dying.

—*Bob Dylan*

Four in the morning and I awoke with a shot. A shot in my chest. An incredibly painful shot in my chest, sudden and penetrating, preventing any movement.

"Oh, my God!" I thought. "A heart attack!" Sweat oozed from all pores, sticking me to the mattress. Just like the stories you hear everyday—healthy young man in his forties keels over from unexpected massive heart trauma. There I was, dying alone in a hotel room, far from home.

Many of us have had a situation in which the fear of death has raised its frightening head. And in the predawn hours the sudden crisis seems to bring the shadow of death even closer. I had always thought at times like this my mind would drop its superficial chatter and focus on the important things—like friends and loved ones and God. Instead, I kept having images of the host of the next morning's conference announcing, "We are sorry but the keynote presentation on stress management has

181

9

been canceled, due to the stress-related death of the speaker."

How could I entertain such thoughts at a time like this? Not only was I dying, but I was feeling guilty about how I was dying! Can't a guy even die without feeling inadequate?

More weird thoughts followed: Maybe it's just something I ate—ouch! No—it's too sharp and high in my chest. Am I dying or what? Maybe I rolled over on something sharp in my sleep? How hot was that sauce at dinner? I can't call the hospital unless I'm sure its serious; I don't want to be tubed up and wheeled around if I only have gas. Maybe I just pulled a—owww! Could this be *it?*

My heart pounded like a drumroll in Arlington Cemetery. It's interesting how uncentered we can become faced with the awareness that we might die.

It's also revealing how religious we get. Thomas Merton once said, "Our idea of God tells us more about ourselves than about Him." Maybe my problem was that I had grown up with too many religions to choose from, leaving only confusion and doubt to spring up from the theological compost. The benefit of blind faith was not mine. The Judeo-Christian notion of heaven and hell gave me considerable trepidation. Hell was terrifying, and I wasn't sure if I fit the criteria for heaven. And, besides, my head was filled with those silly, trite, pastoral images of white robes and harpists, not exactly the environment I would choose under normal circumstances.

Another sharp pain, another confused thought. Hey, maybe reincarnation was a possibility. But it would be a struggle to get into a seven-pound ten-ounce (hopefully human) body again. The prospect of a new body with healthy knees was exciting, but what if I screwed it up all over again? And was I so important that recycling me was automatic? I had my doubts.

I gingerly turned onto my side in search of comfort. So what about existentialism? But that left me with only the prospect of nothingness, the absolute void, the deep sleep with no awakening. Better than the inferno surely, as it came with a guarantee of pain-free nonexistence.

There I was in the wee hours, dying alone in my hotel room and frantically shopping around for the best religion. As the great neurotic Woody Allen said, "How can I find meaning in a finite universe given my shirt and waist size?" Something told me I'd better embrace them all. No sense going for the wrong pitch when it's a three and two count in the bottom of the ninth.

But maybe not. In the end, aren't Christians, Jews, Muslims, Buddhists, Hindus, and the occasional Druid all staring down the same gun barrel? Or is that a tunnel? *Breathe.*

If I was going to get a handle on the chaos in my mind, I needed to get centered. I struggled my way to a seated position against the bed board. I breathed deeply and closed my eyes. Crazy thoughts continued . . . I wondered if, when they discovered me dead, I'd still be in this meditative state, serene and angelic? Maybe I should get dressed, brush my hair, and die looking good, following Woody Allen's infallible logic, "Eternal nothingness is okay if you're dressed appropriately." Breathe . . . Relax and Let God . . . But what if . . . Breathe . . . But . . . Breathe.

Peace is hard to come by when pain and anxiety are running roughshod through the mind. Yet, with each deep breath from center, I began to let go of that clinging, fearful part of me and to relax. I began to hear the sound of raindrops on the windowsill. A simple raindrop. Rising from the ocean, into the heavens, transforming to a drop of moisture, bouncing off the windowsill, joining some endless stream in the dance back to the ocean.

The ocean ebbed and flowed in my consciousness. It took over my meditation. I began to let go of the part of me that was the raindrop and became intoxicated with the unbounded ocean. Why hang on to the drop, struggling to perpetuate it, when the ocean was so much more enticing? Its soft unboundedness and mystery somehow bathed me in comfort.

The poet monk Nanpaku wrote:

Quite apart from our religion
There are plum blossoms.
There are cherry blossoms.

And Walt Whitman, in *Leaves of Grass,* concurred: "Now I re-examine philosophies and religions. They may prove well in lecture-rooms, yet not prove at all under the spacious clouds and along the landscape and flowing currents."

And in the Mysterious Ocean, filled with waves of life and death . . . But what if . . . Breathe, breathe in the Mystery. . . . But what difference would it make if I went to heaven, simply returned to the elements, or came back with a new body? . . . Breathe. . . . It wouldn't change how I lived. True happiness still only comes from loving, compassionate service to life. . . . Breathe. . . . But . . . breathe . . . breathe in the Mystery . . . But if I could live in this Mystery continuously, I would infuse every moment with spirit. . . . Only in the Mystery is absolutely security. . . . Breathe. . . .

I slowly opened my eyes. It was 5:05 A.M. I felt like I had been sitting there for hours. My mind was clearer. I felt some pain, but I was more comfortable with it. I located the phone on the nightstand and managed to call the emergency room.

"I hate to bother you, but I have some questions concerning heart attacks," I said, sounding as academic as possible, like I was writing a research paper.

But you can't fool an emergency nurse at 5 A.M. Her response was direct, yet soothing, and I didn't even have to fill out any forms.

"Are you having the problem?"

"Uh, yes. I think so."

Why was I so embarrassed? I relayed my symptoms.

"Does it hurt worse when you palpate the area with your fingers?"

"Yes," I replied definitively after a few pressurized touches.

"That's a good sign. Palpation on the chest usually doesn't increase the pain in a heart attack."

Whew! I've never heard more freeing words. Palpation, my new mantra. Bluebirds appeared on my shoulder, zippety-do-dahs in my mind. I wasn't dying! The sun would rise again.

I thanked the nurse so profusely for her assistance that she had difficulty accepting the adulation. Then I settled back into meditation, a meditation of thanks and more palpations.

At 7 A.M. my other wake-up call came. I couldn't move from side to side. It was torture to sit up. And I couldn't have been happier. What's a little pain? I smiled as I crawled to the shower. An hour later I was putting massive amounts of Ben-Gay on the area and visualizing myself doing my aikido demo from center, fluidly and gracefully.

The seminar went beautifully. No sharp cries, or dramatic death-falls into the audience. Before the demonstration I mentioned to my assistant Rod O'Connor that I was suffering from a chest injury, possibly a torn rib cartilage, but that I would be fine for the job we had to do.

"You're awfully happy for an injured guy," he observed.

It was an insightful lesson in the principle of contrast. Almost Gone, real or imagined, made me more alive than the most restful night ever would have done.

An old African Bushman once said that "the white man doesn't have a shadow." Could it be that until we accept the Shadow, we will never learn how to walk joyfully on this earth?

One of my heroes and mentors, Buckminster Fuller, had an Almost Gone experience of a different nature. His story has inspired me often.

We tend to consider that this great thinker, mathematician,

185

and inventor, with thousands of patents to his name, including the geodesic dome, must have always had his act together. Nothing could be further from the truth. Bucky himself would be the first to tell you that he took quite an arduous path to finding himself.

Coming from a long lineage of Harvard alumni, it was assumed that young Bucky would go to Harvard. Apparently no one checked with Bucky about his own wishes. During his first semester at Harvard, Bucky hung out in New York City, spending his entire tuition allowance entertaining women and partying. After he was "dismissed" from Harvard, he worked with a cotton mill in Canada, helping it become more productive through his creative ideas and innovations. Because of his success, his family and Harvard strongly "encouraged" him to return to school. Proving that you cannot always get it right the second time, he once more repeated the Broadway binge and was again given the boot. When Bucky told me this story, it seemed incongruous to listen to this deeply compassionate and wise grandfather of eighty-three talk about youthful debauchery.

One foolish mistake followed another. He went into a building business for money, not love. It took time for Bucky to realize that not following your heart and your passion is to swim upstream against the flow of life. As we often do when we are in a business for the wrong reasons, Bucky demonstrated that he was a consummate failure, at least to himself. Driven to drink, he periodically escaped from his painful life in New York by returning to the Harvard campus for nights of drunkenness. Yet Bucky had a reason to hang in there—his deep love for his wife Annie and their little four-year-old daughter Alexandra.

One morning, just before Bucky headed off for another weekend spree, he found himself by his daughter's bedside. As he hugged her good-bye, she asked Bucky for a favor. She was very ill. Would he bring a Harvard pennant for her when he came back? She just loved the pennants with their colorful flags and sturdy, smooth wooden handles.

"Of course," Bucky had responded to his precious daughter.

Three days later Bucky was still at Harvard, hung over from a weekend of debauchery, when he received an emergency call from home. His daughter was critically ill. Pulling himself together, he rushed to the train station.

A few hours later he arrived home and sat by Alexandra's side, taking her tiny hand into his. She looked up at him with a weak smile and said, "Did you have fun, Daddy?"

"Yes, darling, I did."

"Did you bring me my pennant?"

Bucky's heart broke. He had forgotten.

His daughter, Alexandra, died soon after.

That broken promise, a small but essential gift forgotten, was like a spear piercing the toughest armor. Bucky was now not only a failure, but he had even let down the one he loved the most. He fell into a downward spiral of despair, heightened by business failure and fueled by alcohol. In his mind he was doing more harm by being alive. Suicide at least would prevent him from doing further harm to others.

Standing over Lake Michigan on a dreary, dark day with the deep, black water beckoning his soul, Bucky prepared to take his life.

What kind of a human being must I be to let down those I love the most? Must I once more waste away my talents and reject the love offered by others?

But as he stared into the blackness from a depth far below his pain, a revelation burst forth. Why waste the most precious gift that he was given—his own life—in order to hide from his pain? Could he not summon the courage to commit another kind of suicide, one which would be far more valuable than sidewalk splattering or bridge dropping. Why not drown only those aspects of himself that were not of service? Why not dedicate his life to becoming a humble servant of the universe?

The transformation of Buckminster Fuller did not happen overnight. He recognized that even his conscious thoughts emerged through the filters of beliefs that he had acquired, and that those cluttered beliefs kept him from discovering who he was. He committed himself to silence until the words that came forth were from a deeper place of truth than the mental garbage that he had carried with him to that point. In a Chicago tenement with his wife Annie, Bucky remained silent for two years before he finally discovered something to say that came from him rather than from the normative system in which he was born and lived. Then, after over three decades of living, Bucky began a new life as a true servant of the universe, basking in its magnificence and sharing some of its basic principles with the rest of the world.

Almost Gone hadn't been a physical illness for Bucky. It had been a mental and emotional one. But Bucky had the courage to come back, not as a selfish little man sucking life dry and complaining about his fate, but as a gift to the future, redefining what it is to be human:

"At present I am a passenger on Spaceship Earth." On the other hand, "I don't know what I am. I know that I am not a category, a highbred specialization. I am not a thing—a noun. I am not flesh. At eighty-five, I have taken in over a thousand tons of air, food, and water, which temporarily became my flesh and which progressively disassociated from me. You and I seem to be verbs—evolutionary processes. Are we not integral functions of the Universe?"

"It will not be a matter of earning a living. You'll be doing what you see needs to be done because you'll feel you'll want to do it—you'll want to qualify to be able to serve one another. . . ."

If you can do it, if it is spontaneously arousable in you to operate with integrity and really go along to love, to love comprehensively, that's it."

A friend of mine, who goes by the unusual name of W. Mitchell, was Almost Gone twice. W. Mitchell was a fun-loving and athletic man who enjoyed the rugged environs and all the physical activities they offered—hiking and biking in the summer, skiing in the winter. One day, while riding his motorcycle to work in San Francisco, he was surprised by a large laundry truck pulling out on the road in front of him. Mitchell had to jam hard on the brakes. He turned sharply to avoid collision, but the slippery pavement caused his bike to skid out from under him, and man and bike slid together underneath the fully loaded truck. The friction from the slide ignited the spilling gasoline and a fire exploded around him. Mercifully, his life was spared, but Mitchell was burned severely over most of his body. He lost most of his face and his hands, leaving massive scar tissue, and stubs for fingers. After numerous surgeries and procedures and months of rehabilitation, Mitchell was back on his feet again, jumping into life with enthusiasm and commitment. Without fingers and with a greatly disfigured face, Mitchell started a successful business and learned to fly an airplane.

One day he was forced to make an emergency landing because of a mechanical failure in the aircraft. He managed to land the plane safely so that none of his passengers was seriously injured. Except for Mitchell. He was paralyzed from the waist down. No fingers, no face, and now no use of legs.

Mitchell chose to appreciate the life he was given and to make the most of it. Sure, there was pain and plenty of it. But Mitchell knew that there was a distinction between pain and suffering. Pain, like joy, comes with life. It is part of life. But suffering, that's a choice. Mitchell still had a choice about how he related to his pain. He could suffer from it, or he could use it as an opportunity to change, to grow, and to take action more effectively.

One day during rehabilitation Mitchell saw a young man alone in his wheelchair, head downcast with depression. The man had been a skier, a mountain biker, and a climber. All those things were now unavailable to him. In his mind his life was finished. Mitchell rolled his wheelchair over to the young man.

"When I was first paralyzed," he said with compassion, "I thought that I was through. Life wasn't worth living. But after a while I realized that before my accidents there were at least ten thousand things I could do. Now there are only nine thousand. I could feel bad about the one thousand things I can't do. Or I could focus on the nine thousand that are still left. And if I could do only two hundred of these, I'd probably be the most productive and happy man on the planet."

Since those days, Mitchell has become a millionaire business-man, married a beautiful woman, been elected mayor of Crested Butte (running under the slogan "Not Just Another Pretty Face"), been a talk-show host, and a pilot once more. I sometimes see Mitchell in airports going to make his inspirational speeches or rafting down the Grand Canyon. Not too long ago he flew me in his plane from San Diego to Aspen. And he did it all with his fingerless hands.

In 1979, Sally Ranney (president of the American Wilderness Alliance), John Denver, and I, representing the Windstar Foundation (an environmental education organization), were presenting a gift to President Carter commemorating his successful work on the Alaska Wildlands bill. Prior to our presentation I was walking through the White House library. There was Mitchell sitting in his wheelchair and reading a book.

"Mitchell, what in the world are you doing here in the White House?"

He looked at me and grinned, "When you look like I do, you can damn near go anywhere you want."

Mitchell, Almost Gone twice, is simply going higher and higher.

*Faith is the bird that sings when
the dawn is still dark.*

—RABINDRANATH TAGORE

APPRECIATE THE MYSTERY

In the warm sunshine it is easy to sit like the Buddha. But when the cold and darkness creep in, carrying a great storm, the test of your convictions begins. And when that great approaching darkness is death, it reveals more about how you have lived than where you are going, more about who you are *now* than who you are becoming. If you think that you will lose your inner peace in those moments, and become a victim, paralyzed by fear, enraged by life's injustices, perhaps there is work to be done.

And what is this work? It is knowing at the deepest level who you are and what your relationship is with the universe. This is centered awareness.

Stephen Levine, who has written numerous books that shed light on the dying process, writes in *Meetings at the Edge:*

. . . We come to the mind's edge, past seemingly solid fears and long-conditioned doubt, and enter the heart of the mystery. Love is the bridge.

This is a high-wire act. To keep the heart open in hell, to maintain some loving balance in the face of all our pain and confusion. To allow life in. To heal past our fear of the unknown.

There is a dramatic difference between this depth of inner

knowing and a superficial declaration of a religious belief. When a belief has not reached the level of knowing, there will be a tendency to become angry or upset when the belief is challenged. For example, if you repeatedly release an apple from your hand, you will eventually know that apples go down, not up, every time (unless you're trying this on the space shuttle). If someone declares that "apples go up," notice that you don't attack them for such blasphemy. Instead, you are fascinated, curious, intent to learn more. This is "knowing."

Knowing who you are brings an inner peace and a nonviolent, compassionate perspective to the unexpected happenings in life, including the loss of a possession, a friend, *or* yourself.

You can develop centered awareness through daily practice. Going inside daily—in meditation, in contemplative prayer, in solitude, in communion with nature—brings clarity to your purpose, your gifts, and your passion. It also brings you face-to-face with your fears and vulnerabilities as, in quiet awareness, you incrementally engage the light side *and* the shadow side, subtly preparing not just for vital living, but also for your eventual death. When your final breaths come, you can accept the Mystery graciously, knowing the impermanence of the body and the eternal nature of consciousness.

When the great darkness blocks out the sun, centered awareness will provide the calm courage to embrace the Mystery. And if you are blessed with another sunrise, your choosing to connect daily with the mystery will enlighten everything—a cup of tea, a stand of trees, a simple hello.

Gone

My barn having burned
to the ground
I can now see
the moon

—JAPANESE HAIKU

The screams startled me out of my slumber. I sat up on the river rock on which I had been sunning myself reptilelike, and squinted through the sun.

"Help! Please help!"

The frantic shouts came from the base of the cliffs. I had seen some climbers with ropes working their way up the cliff earlier. I jammed my feet in my tennis shoes and began clambering over the boulders. I leaped onto soft earth and sprinted up the hill.

In the distance, I could see ropes scattered about and two people hovering over something on the ground. Their movements appeared sudden, frantic. As I got closer, it became clear that the men were administering CPR to another man—a young man in his early twenties, muscular and lean. He was bleeding from his mouth, nose, and ears, and his legs were twitching beyond control.

But, as I watched, the twitching of his legs began to quiet

9

down. His fingers, which kept grasping the air as if trying to find something to hold on to, suddenly lay still.

"Come on! Don't give up!" shouted his friend over him.

The injured man's chest suddenly heaved, his eyes shot open, and he began to scream. "Oh God, oh God. Mother, please help me. Help me!"

A passing vehicle was summoned to get mountain rescue help from Aspen. I looked at my watch. Medical help wouldn't be here for at least forty-five minutes. I kept looking at the man's young, grasping hands. I knelt down and placed my hand in his grasp and I put my other one on his forehead.

"Just keep breathing deep," I offered. "Medical help is on the way."

Another shot of pain coursed through his body.

"Oh God. Please. Mother! Help me."

He lapsed back into unconsciousness. Again there was no sign of breathing. His friends began in earnest, one trying to pump life into his chest, the other breathing his own life into the man's mouth.

One of the men looked up to the cliff, shook his head, and said to no one in particular, "He fell so far."

I looked up. The ledge was about a hundred feet above us. I shivered at the thought. The steepness of the cliff suggested it was a free fall to the rocks below.

Suddenly, he was breathing again, his eyes wide open. He began to cry, tears flowing down his cheeks into the blood-stained dirt where he lay. Written across his innocent, wrinkle-free face in a pleading, terrified look were the unspoken words "Get me out of this nightmare!"

His face brought tears to mine. I had a question too. Why him? Why? Just hours earlier he must have been full of youthful hopes and dreams and a myriad of mundane thoughts. Now he desperately wanted simply to live. Just as suddenly as the life force brought him awake, it would leave. We pressed on with

194

prayerful thoughts, and CPR. And, after a few moments, the vacant eyes would magically fill with life. Spirit would somehow reenter this human container that we held. At times, he seemed to be more at peace than before, his eyes less panicked and fearful, as if he had received some knowledge on his brief trips outside the body. For the next forty-five minutes, even after the mountain rescue folks had arrived at the scene, this life force would come and go.

"Giving up the ghost" had real meaning for the first time. The man in my hands weighed the same, looked the same. But that spirit which gave him life, made him who he was, was invisible, weightless, outside of form. When "It" finally left the body for good there was no doubt, and everyone felt it.

To be able to watch and touch the ebb and flow of life had been an honor. To have it happen so painfully, so fearfully, so unexpectedly, so helplessly, in the prime of youth, tore at our guts, and twisted us inside. Why? Why him? And what is this life that courses through our bodies one moment and then leaves it, letting it rot the next? It was the first time I had watched a human die. It wasn't pretty, it was painful, and there was nothing we could do about it.

> *Dew evaporates*
> *and all our world*
> *is dew . . . so dear*
> *so refreshing, so fleeting*
> *This dewdrop world*
> *It may be dewdrop*
> *And yet . . . and yet . . .*

—ISSA, ON THE DEATH OF HIS CHILD

195

Years later, I heard a knock at our door on a warm summer evening. I studied his face as he entered. It was Ralph Jackson, Aspen's legendary ski bum. He didn't have on the signature top hat and full-length raccoon coat with the tails in which he had performed his acrobatic ski antics practically every winter day since Aspen became a ski town. He had been a fixture around Aspen long before most of the locals had even thought about moving to Colorado. With each year his face gathered a few more wrinkles, his hair and whiskers grew a little more gray, and his skiing became a little less outrageous. But the twinkle in his eye never diminished, nor his leering wink at the ladies, nor the quantity of spirits in his flask. A pretty woman to flirt with, a quick slug from his flask, a little backward skiing, and he was a happy man.

Ralph lived alone, down the block from us, in an old shack reminiscent of the mining days. We would pass on the street, me riding my bike, he out for his daily walk, sporting his cane. I'd say, "Hi, Ralph! How goes it?" and he'd mumble some line that may have been funny if I could have understood it, but he talked in a deep, gravelly voice that slipped out of one corner of his mouth as if the other side was sewn shut. But the twinkle in his eye did the real speaking—he liked my family and me, and wasn't life a huge joke?

"Ralph!" Cathy welcomed him. This was a unique occurrence. Cathy had always thought that for all his gregarious ways, Ralph had no close friends. About a year prior, she had invited him to come over to our house if he ever "needed anything." But he never did.

"Hey, how ya doin'," he muttered. Then he looked directly at me, which he didn't usually do.

"Mind if I come in and sit with you folks a spell?"

"Oh, please do!" Cathy said. "Would you like some tea, or lemonade, or something?"

"Thanks."

He collapsed in an armchair by the window.

"I'm not feelin' too well," he mumbled. "Nice day though."

I got the feeling that Ralph's twinkle came from years of practice. He had it down, even when things weren't going so well.

"Are you all right, Ralph? What's the matter?"

"Oh, it's nothing. Little pain in the chest. Some difficulty breathing. I think it musta been something I ate. Probably that chili."

Now Ralph was a crusty old coot. We all knew that he knew it was more serious than that.

"Ralph, why don't we take you up to the hospital. This could be serious."

He looked me straight in the eye.

"Nope. I'll have none of that nonsense. Tubes down my throat, needles in my arm, hooked up to all kinds of metal contraptions. No, it's just indigestion. I just want to stay here with you folks, if you know what I mean."

We knew what he meant. And, the truth was, it felt right not to take him to the hospital.

Cathy brought the tea. Ralph looked tired, but the twinkle hadn't left completely. He started telling jokes again, one-liners interlaced with comments like, "If I make it through this, I'm gonna write a book. That's what I'll do. Write a book."

After tea I asked if we could massage him a bit, hoping that some kiatsu and body work would help. Cathy and I teamed up, I worked on his arms and Cathy on his shoulders, neck and back. He loved it.

"I'm gonna have to eat that chili more often," he wisecracked.

He asked if he could lie down to rest. He didn't want a bed, he just wanted the living room floor. Cathy fetched a blanket and pillow and he stretched out on the rug. I suggested that he breathe deep and full, which he did. It was then that I noticed he wasn't wearing his false teeth.

197

9

A half hour later he felt much better, the biggest indicator being his return to off-color one-liners that you could barely decipher, curling his lips around his gums as he chuckled in response. I became more and more inspired by this old man's ability to be so full of humor and without complaint, knowing very well that he may be breathing his last breath, content simply to be with some fellow human beings.

This man had come over to die, as simply as if he had dropped by to borrow a cup of sugar.

Cathy and I both knew the situation we were in. If Ralph really was choosing to die here, then what a courageous way to do it. He was molding an environment with his wit and his grit, allowing Cathy and me to be at peace ourselves. The fact that we didn't insist on taking Ralph to the hospital placed us in a precarious position. But we didn't even question it. That he had somehow chosen us to share in his passage was a gift, and we accepted it.

About 6 A.M. Cathy woke me.

"I think it's over," she whispered.

I went in and looked at Ralph. He looked as peaceful as a newborn, just as when we'd said good night, with one exception. No breathing. By his side lay his crooked wooden cane, a vaudevillian symbol of his strength and humor.

And there was one other exception. His false teeth were back in his mouth.

We called the hospital to report the death. Then we sat in deep peace and prayer beside Ralph. But within minutes paramedics were in my living room, shouting orders to each other and piercing the peaceful environment with quick, frenzied movements, resuscitators, assorted equipment. One began a frantic CPR on Ralph's vacated body. His first pushing movements were so strong I thought I heard a rib breaking in Ralph's chest.

"I think he passed on some time ago," Cathy told them quietly.

They didn't respond, so frenzied were they, and intent upon revival. We knew they were just doing their job. They were responding to an emergency call in an emergency way. They had not been in the house all evening like we had been, hanging out with a man willing to be fully present and embrace his death with dignity and lightness. I looked at the body that the medics were trying to kick-start back to life. This was the second death I had "participated" in, and it was much different. Or I was. This time it had occurred peacefully, by choice. I felt Ralph's spirit somewhere in the room, wisecracking with a little chuckle and that sandpaper voice, delivered out of the corner of his mouth, "See what I mean about the hospital? Next they'll be jamming some tubes down my throat. A slug of whiskey would have been a lot cheaper."

One evening I found myself at a conference in Washington, D.C. And as fate would have it, Bucky Fuller happened to be making a presentation that evening at another conference in the very same hotel. I got to the ballroom in time to hear the end of Bucky's lecture. I was in awe of this little man in his eighties, with his clear mind, deep wisdom, and boundless energy. At the end of the talk we walked together through the underground parking lot to his airport limousine.

"I've got to go to New York City tonight for another presentation," he said, looking at me with an anxiousness that I had rarely seen in Bucky.

"You know, Annie's not doing well. I'm very concerned about her."

We hugged.

Bucky Fuller had once confided to me that he had promised his wife Annie to die before her, so that he could be there to welcome her when it was her turn. I took the comment as a

199

hope, not a commitment. Which shows how greatly I underestimated Buckminster Fuller.

Shortly after Bucky's presentation in New York, he was informed that Annie had lapsed into a coma in a hospital in Los Angeles. Doctors felt that there was a good chance she would not regain consciousness. Bucky took the first flight he could get. Upon arriving in Los Angeles, he went immediately to Annie's bedside. Sitting beside her, he closed his eyes.

And quietly died.

The power to choose life fully was something that Bucky exemplified. So much so that he had the power to choose death when it was time, peacefully, with arms wide open to the universe that he served. It was simply another courageous step forward.

Hours later Annie peacefully joined him in death. He had kept his promise; he was waiting for her.

Jack Boland, a friend of mine and beloved minister to thousands in the Detroit area, also chose to accept death with dignity, courage, and humor. Always a man of flair and charisma, he certainly did not want to miss the celebration of his own death. He got permission from his physicians to leave his hospital bed and be wheeled into his Church of Today chapel during Sunday service, where he had assembled his closest friends from throughout the world and delivered his own eulogy. His once-strong voice weakened with cancer, he struggled from the wheelchair to deliver an inspirational sermon, asking the congregation to keep lit the flame of the church.

He quoted the dying words spoken by a fellow patriot, John Quincy Adams: "John Quincy Adams is well. It's just the house in which he lives that's falling apart. He may have to move out of it soon. That's all. But John Quincy Adams is well, quite well."

Shortly thereafter, a mutual friend, Christophe Dean, was sitting alone by Jack's bedside. Jack had been going in and out of consciousness. He had been receiving people all week, filling each with inspiration and love. An aura of peace surrounded him. Slowly, he opened his eyes and looked at Christophe and smiled.

"Can you imagine the apologies I'll have to make if I don't die?"

He closed his eyes again. More time passed, and then he slowly opened them again and, with a deep look of happiness, uttered the last words that Christophe heard him speak: "Can you believe this?"

> *Sixty-six times have these eyes beheld*
> *the changing scenes of Autumn*
> *I have said enough about moonlight,*
> *Ask me no more.*
> *Only listen to the voice of pines and cedars,*
> *when no wind stirs.*

—RYO-NEN (HER LAST COMPOSITION)

LET GO, LET GOD

With the ego at the helm we let ourselves be defined by our possessions, our professions, our relationships, our beliefs. As tough as it is to let go of our attachment to these, it's easy in comparison to our excessive identification with the body. Hence our preoccupation with death.

The young man who fell from the cliff was jarred suddenly into facing his attachment to life. The suffering and pain was intense, and the frantic grasping of his hands reflected his desperate clinging.

In contrast, Ralph Jackson's passage was peaceful and accepting. He followed his own unique path through life, letting go of the societal pressures to become a ski bum long before the idea was popularized. This adventurous spirit and courage to stand alone served him well in the end. To his final breath he lived Santayana's words, "There is no cure for birth and death, save to enjoy the interval."

Likewise, Bucky Fuller challenged conventional wisdom his entire life. His relentlessly penetrating, inquiring mind connected him deeply with what he called the "Integrity of Universe," enabling him to participate consciously in choosing the moment of his death.

And Jack Boland smiled his way into death because of his great faith. When he was young, a bout with alcoholism had taught him that he couldn't do it alone. After years of ministering to thousands, he learned that in truth he is never alone. Even the passage from this life could be guided with love every step.

It takes an adventurous spirit to give up the attachment to the body and step willingly into the unknown. It assumes a fundamental desire to discover and to serve, and a deep trust in a principled universe.

And what is death anyway? Could it be that our understanding is still at a developmental stage, as when we believed the world was flat and that the earth was the center of the universe?

To most of us, our concept of death is based on the "common-sense," subjective experience of linear time. Let's say we draw a line on a blackboard delineating time. The left endpoint would dictate our date of birth and a series of dates and dots along the line would mark various events until we get to a final dot on the right side to indicate death. We should have no problem understanding this time line of life because it follows conventional wisdom about how time flows from past through present to future. But what if this is just a naive understanding of the universe, as some of our cutting edge thinkers are proposing?

Larry Dossey, M.D., in his seminal book *Space, Time, and Medicine*, brings forth many findings from modern scientists, mathematicians, and physicists to declare that science has shown for many years that linear time and even our conceptual death as a culminating endpoint is purely subjective. Physicist-mathematician P. C. W. Davies states, "No physical experiment has ever been performed that detects the passage of time." And the late German mathematician Hermann Weyl concurs: "The world doesn't happen, it simply is."

Dossey's work gives us much to consider. It suggests that the one-way flow of linear time does not exist other than in our minds. Further, modern science tells us that we can't put "boundaries" on time, nor on our constantly changing and recycling bodies. Therefore, there is logically no "beginning point" called birth or "ending point" called death. As Einstein said about a friend's death, "This signifies nothing. For us believing physicists the distinction between past, present, and future is only an illusion, even if a stubborn one."

Are we embarking on a new Copernican-like revolution concerning the issue of death and the passage of time? And what lessons from our past could support us on this voyage?

The natives of Patagonia could only see the little rowboats from Darwin's ship and entirely missed seeing Darwin's huge mother ship, the *Beagle,* because their model of reality only allowed them to see little canoes like their own. Could it be as difficult for us to "see" such challenging thoughts as "there is no past, present, and future" or "death does not exist as an end, or boundary, to life"? Perhaps, the Mother Ship is out there now, just waiting to be seen.

Attempting to understand the nature of death is an ideological and evolutionary endeavor. Perhaps more rewarding than our theorizing is our ability to appreciate life's Mystery. It can be a great gift to truly *be* with friends and relatives when they are dying, or to volunteer at a hospice—a blessing for you as well as for those departing. In generations past, people grew up watching the birth and

203

9

death of many in their village, learning that life is both precious and cyclical. When you enter new frontiers with centered awareness and an open, discovering spirit, great vitality and freedom is possible. Just imagine what is awaiting you if you enter the Great Mystery with those same qualities.

The Warrior Spirit

Uncentered we hide
Scared of the Shadow
Piling up stories, brick by brick

Some years back I was asked to make a presentation on commitment at the annual Windstar Symposium. It was a Saturday night gathering, with an audience of about fifteen hundred enthusiastic people who had already spent two full days in workshops. For the most part, they were already committed to making a difference in the world. Like most successful people, they knew the importance of purpose and vision. But could they manifest their visions?

We all know how companies send their management teams on retreat in a nice resort and spend several days to become crystal clear about the organizational vision and then return with a commitment to align their employees around it. As individuals, we go to workshops ourselves and return home rejuvenated and ready. The vision statements appear on our bulletin boards at work or in our personal journals, and we all get pumped up. For about two weeks. Or maybe six months. But often, the statements just kind of fade out of the picture. Why? That was what I wanted to get at.

I proposed that most people and organizations lack the warrior spirit. "To live fully, one must be willing to die" is a samurai maxim that enables a warrior to be aware and present and powerful in battle. Most of us aren't strapping on metal swords each day. Yet, we all have a certain affinity with the concept of warrior. The word "warrior" itself evokes images of honor, courage, honesty, loyalty, and service. But the aspects of the warrior are diluted today. Modern warfare, Hollywood movies, and TV bring out needless aggression, brutality, and insensitivity. They clutter the picture of the true warrior.

I gave the audience my definition of a warrior:

"A true warrior today must each moment cut through his story, and step forth from his vision. Each moment the true warrior must cut through her story, and step forth from her vision."

Though I'm sure they appreciated my stab at political correctness, they had no idea what I was talking about. So I selected a big, strong volunteer named Steve from the audience. Steve was to represent "my story." Our stories might be a bad cold, not being young or old enough, not wanting to rock the boat, or any number of things that convince us to believe "I can't do this." I asked Steve to grab me from behind in a bear hug to keep me from walking forward, which he did easily. Then I asked the audience to watch several scenarios.

In the first situation we demonstrated how ridiculously easy it was for him to keep me motionless if I had nowhere to go. At the first little sign of resistance I would give up the struggle to go forward. In the second scenario I held a purpose and vision in my mind and put it out in front of me across the stage. I made sure that it was something that was vivid and compelling and important. My neck strained forward and I was in a tug-of-war between the direction that I wanted to go and the resistance of the arms around my chest. I made some headway, demonstrating a lot more power and enthusiasm than in the first scenario, and yet he was still able to hold me back.

"You can see that purpose and vision are important," I said to the audience. "They give me more power. But somehow they aren't enough. What keeps me back is not my lack of purpose. It is my story."

Stories are legitimate or illegitimate considerations that grab our minds and our bodies and hold us back. For instance, if a young girl sings a song in front of her parents and is met with laughter and jeers, she may become trapped in the story: "I'm not good enough to be a singer." It is unlikely that she will audition for a play, even if theater is her passion. And, if she is required to, her willingness to bring forth her best will be held back, entrapped in her story just as strongly as I was in Steve's grasp.

We tend to operate out of our stories, rather than from our center. In my case this big guy with his arms around me represented my story—a rather large and compelling story at that—and two times he had held me back.

In the third scenario, I suggested to the audience that whether our stories are real or imagined, they are real for us. Instead of denying their existence, we've got to accept them, thank them for their lessons, and then get on with our vision. But it must be done from center, not story. To demonstrate this I stepped back (rather than struggling to go forward) acknowledging Steve's strength and reestablishing my center. From this centered place I moved powerfully forward from center with my mind and body extended as one unit of energy toward my vision. Instead of straining from the chest area where his arms were, as I had done in the second attempt, I literally moved from my center. I accepted the story, but did not operate from it. In this case my story was a large man named Steve, whom I was effortlessly dragging behind me. But it could have been anything people allow to get them off center, from rush-hour traffic

207

to a disagreement with their spouse. When I did this, the audience could see that I was walking across the stage with power and grace, and there just happened to be this big appendage hanging on.

And "hanging on" is just too hard in the face of centered movement. Steve eventually would have to make a choice; either walk with me or let go and go his own way. Stories have a way of doing just that. Good leadership is similar. The best leaders don't have to coerce, carry, or manipulate people. They simply have to live their lives with congruency of love, purpose, and action. When they do this, their teammates will show up because they are able to recognize that clear direction as theirs also, and as a result will accept responsibility for their own steps along the way.

The difference in power between moving from center and the first two attempts was vivid to the audience. As long as we operate out of our stories, we are far less alive and powerful regardless of how great our visions are. But to center ourselves, and to accept and not deny our stories, is to learn from them. When we take action, we do so from our centered vision.

That's the true warrior spirit.

If you're not centered in your vision, it is easy to get caught up in your stories. In the heat of the battle it's easy to let your story speak loudly in counterproductive ways.

"I'm not cultured enough."

"I'm too emotional."

"My father expected too much of me."

"I was an only child."

"My parents wanted me to be a boy."

"I have a chronic knee problem."

208

Do you notice how our stories are always just good enough to justify why we don't get our expectations met? If all you need is a cold to keep you down, you get a cold. If you need a Mack truck to run you over, you get that. Have you ever noticed that when two people sit down and start talking about their lives that their "stories" are just good enough to justify where they find themselves at that moment?

"The reason my life is such a mess," Bill cries into his beer, "is that I grew up in a dysfunctional family, my dad was an alcoholic, my sister got all the accolades, my brother tried to drown me in the bathtub, and a hippopotamus rolled over me when I was sleeping."

Some are true, some are exaggerated, some are imagined. As long as the person "feels" it on his back, it's on his back. And with each new story he gets to play the victim a little more, further justifying why he is not living out his vision.

"I'm not smart enough. I'm not young enough. I'm not the right color. I'm not wealthy enough." The list goes on and on, doesn't it?

These stories are likely to take over, especially under pressure, unless you have a centered vision that you can turn to for power and focus. It is the daily practice of center and centered purpose that brings out the true warrior spirit.

As George Bernard Shaw said,

> This is the true joy in life. The being used for a purpose recognized by yourself as a mighty one; the being thoroughly worn out before you are thrown on the scrap heap, the being a force of nature instead of a feverish, selfish little clod of ailments and grievances, complaining that the world will not devote itself to making you happy.

When a group of people get centered together around a vision, mountains move. Charles Garfield, one of tens of thousands of scientists in the 1960s working on the Apollo XI mission, explains:

I was trained as a mathematician, and was going to be a scientist. With that in mind, I joined a team involved in realizing what is generally regarded as one of the human species' greatest technological achievements—the Apollo XI mission to the moon.

From my first day on that job, I started hearing stories of people doing the best work in their lives, better work than they had ever done before. I later found, as part of the assessment team, that we were talking about tens of thousands of people, not just a few. I asked why, but nobody could tell me. So I kept trying to figure it out. In multiple facilities around the United States, workers averaged thirty to forty percent increases in productivity. Adequate-to-good performers were suddenly doing great work. Yet we were paid poorly, and the work conditions were lousy. Why were so many people doing the best work in their lives? I had no idea, and nobody else seemed to know why, either.

One day, out of frustration, I grabbed my boss, who was trained as an engineer. I asked him, "George, what's going on here?" George pulled me out into the parking lot—it was early evening—and said, "Look, kid, you want to know why so many people are doing the best work in their lives? That's the reason"—and he pointed to the moon. He said, "That's the reason. People have been talking about going there for thousands of years, and you and I are going to be a part of making it happen. . . ." Then he used a word that I now think you can take to the bank; he looked at me and said, "You want to know why we're doing so well, Charlie? We've got a mission."

My warrior spirit demonstration of walking from center generated great interest in the audience. But I knew that there would still be a tendency in a certain portion of the audience to say, "Well, that all sounds good. But you haven't heard *my* story yet."

Predicting this, I invited two close friends onstage to share their stories. Both were near the end of long-standing battles with disease. They were poignant and inspirational examples of people who were fueled by their stories, not burdened by them.

Treya Killam Wilber had been a close friend for twenty years. She was Tommy's godmother, and like a sister to Cathy and me. Ten days after marrying the man of her dreams, she found herself on her honeymoon in the hospital with stage-two breast cancer. And now five years later the cancer had metastasized to her brain and lungs and she was dying. Always a stunningly beautiful woman, she was now barely in her forties. And bald. And even more lovely, in the graceful, serene way she moved, and in the light and wisdom that sparkled from her eyes. The five-year battle had at once ravaged her body and strengthened her soul.

During her illness, Treya had not retreated from life. Instead, she had jumped into it with the same brilliance and curiosity she always had. Only this time the subject matter, which used to be skiing and pottery and environmental causes, changed to healing and dying. She created a cancer support center in San Francisco for others in her condition to come together. She personally counseled hundreds of patients, and she began to write regularly to her network of friends throughout the world of her relationship to cancer, its gifts and its lessons, so that others could find value and understanding from her journey. Joined by her husband Ken Wilber, who later wrote of this experience in his book *Grace and Grit,* she shared her heart and soul, the pain and fear, the joy and hope, the deep depression and even deeper bliss. She even wrote of her experience of the mundane and endless procedures and remedies—from high-tech radiation to coffee enemas.

Many of us gained inspiration, strength, and growth from Treya's letters and visits. Her work became not so much a struggle with cancer by a dying person, as a compassionate practice of

211

a spiritual seeker, an endless reminder that even in sickness and death, as in health and life, we can continue to be centered.

> I had long periods at first when I felt incredibly shaky, crying a lot, very agitated, close to falling apart, dwelling on fears of pain and thoughts of death . . . and then, unbidden, would come thoughts of all who are suffering on this planet at this moment, of all who have suffered in the past, and I would immediately feel a wave of peace and calm pass through me. I no longer felt alone, I no longer felt singled out; instead I felt an incredible connection with all these people, like we were part of the same huge family.
>
> What gives life meaning is helping other people. Service, in a word. Human relationship, human connections, indeed gentle loving relationship with all forms of life and all of creation, only that seems important.

Even her mundane activities took on a heightened awareness of living fully in the moment:

> It's odd to buy a new car with a six-year warranty and wonder if I'll be around when the warranty runs out. It's odd to hear people making plans five years ahead and wonder if I'll be around then. It's odd to think I'd better not put something like terracing the garden off until next year because I may not be around to enjoy it. It's odd to try and explain to the landscaper that I want the rock garden to look lush now so please use big plants, I can't wait three or four years for it to fill in.

212

The process of death and dying can be a strong motivator for exploring center, as Treya demonstrated:

"Surrender to God." Straightforward, direct, composed of what were once two major buzz-words for me. Surrender and God. But now I love it! It's exactly what I need. The shock value, a holdover from what those words once meant to me, wakes me up. It brings me back to mindfulness. I find that when I practice this, when I repeat this phrase, I suddenly let go of whatever was preoccupying me, my awareness opens and expands, and for a moment I suddenly see and feel the beauty and energy all around me, pouring into me, extending out to infinity. And the word God makes me think not of a patriarch but of vastness and emptiness and power and completeness and everlastingness and fullness.

On my drive over, I cried at the sheer majestic beauty of Independence Pass and the next day when I went to my meditation cabin I cried at the simple beauty of the sun shining through aspen leaves. Neither of those moments would have happened if I hadn't been aware I might not be around to see these things year after year. All this beauty makes me so appreciate life that I just can't help but want more and more of it! It's hard not to cling, not to feel attached when I'm surrounded by things like the cleansing sound of a crystal clear stream shaded by tall cottonwoods, when I hear the distinctive soft flutter of a breeze through a stand of quaking aspen trees, when I'm mightily entertained by the bounding gracefulness of critters scurrying through the green undergrowth, when I look up at night and gasp at the unexpected clarity and brightness of myriad stars in a sky that seems suddenly crowded.

213

Treya gave one of the most beautiful definitions of center I have ever heard:

9

It has suddenly occurred to me that our normal understanding of what passion means is loaded with the idea of
clinging, of wanting something or someone, of fearing losing them, of possessiveness. What if you had passion without all that stuff, passion without attachment, passion clean
and pure? What would that be like, what would that mean?
I thought of those moments in meditations when I've felt
my heart open, a painfully wonderful sensation, a passionate feeling but without clinging to any content or person
or thing. And the two words suddenly coupled in my
mind and made a whole. Passionate equanimity, passionate
equanimity—to be fully passionate about all aspects of life,
about our relationship with spirit, to care to the depths of
one's being but with no trace of clinging or holding, that's
what the phrase has come to mean to me. It feels full,
rounded, complete, and challenging.

As Treya stood alone on that stage in front of fifteen hundred
people, wracked and shriveled by the cancer that would take her
life six months hence, I was entranced by her beauty, spirit, and
wisdom. With her heart wide open, she slowly and clearly concluded:

I often find myself in the familiar trap of equating success
with physical healing against all odds or with concrete
accomplishments in the world. I feel instead that what
we're here to celebrate is an inner change. Learning to
make friends with cancer, learning to make friends with
the possibility of an early and perhaps painful death has
taught me a great deal about making friends with myself as
I am and a great deal about making friends with life as it is.
With this growing acceptance of life as it is, with all the
sorrow, pain, and suffering and tragedy, I find myself more

committed to peace. I find myself more connected with all beings that suffer in a more genuine way. And I find a more open sense of compassion and I find a steadier desire to help in whatever way I can. Because I can no longer ignore death, I pay more attention to life.

The audience was silent, deeply moved by Treya's compassionate honesty.

After several minutes of silence Mark Twain stood up from his seat in the audience and solemnly asked if he could take the stage. I accepted, of course, as it was all part of the plan. During the entire three-day symposium, Mark Twain had been in the audience periodically asking questions of the speakers and providing short pieces of wisdom and humor. He was a lively connecting thread.

Mark Twain was actually Bill McLinn, a good friend who had spent the last twelve years touring the world and performing authentic and entertaining one-man shows. Bill had studied Twain's every nuance and speech, his clothing, and his movements, and could mesmerize an audience for hours. And he could do the extraordinary: he could extemporaneously answer questions from the audience on any issue, as Twain, and using Twain's actual words. Mark Twain always had something to say that was bitingly relevant.

What the audience did not know was that Bill/Mark was going to reveal his real story. And, as he had told me earlier, by revealing his story he could very possibly jeopardize everything. His career, his primary relationships, his very life were at stake. And yet, he knew he had to get centered, embrace his story, learn its lessons, and move on toward his vision.

As he walked onto the stage, he was the quintessential Mark Twain. With his turn-of-the-century three-piece suit, his slow gait, his white hair in disarray, he warmed up the audience with

215

a few one-liners on human foibles, and politics in general. But then he grew solemn.

> *I learned people through the heart, not the intellect. I learned that courage is not absence of fear but mastery of fear. I learned that loyalty to petrified opinion has never yet broken a chain or freed a human soul in this world, and never will. I also learned . . . that life is a dream—you, I, we—all are a dream.*

And then, as Twain spoke, he reached up with one hand and peeled off a bushy white eyebrow.

> *Now in this dream I am simply a figment of your imagination.*

Another sentence, and off came the other eyebrow.

> *Nothing exists but you. And even you are a dream.*

With each sentence another piece of Mark Twain was removed—the mustache, the make up, the nineteenth-century jacket. Though he still used Twain's words, it was Bill McLinn who was being revealed.

> *But it gives us the opportunity to dream other dreams and better.*

Twain took off his wig, and in mid-sentence, to the astonishment of the audience, his voice changed from the deeper, gravelly Twain to the softer, more youthful Bill McLinn. Then, as he wiped off the remaining makeup, fifteen hundred people could see the real face behind their lovable Twain. A face discolored with ugly purple blemishes brought on by leukemia-related symptoms associated with the HIV virus. For years he had dispensed with chemotherapy and other harsh treatments that might prevent him from getting out of bed and being Mark Twain. There was a dark shadow upon him.

Bill McLinn then revealed his own story. He had been a theology student who, without formal theatrical training, had astonished his theater professor by stating his intention of putting on a one-man show of Mark Twain.

"Not even seasoned actors would dream of doing a one-man show, let alone Mark Twain."

Bill smiled at the audience.

"But without theater training, I had no context in which to hold his admonitions. So I did it anyway. I found out that people can do anything they want, if they put their mind and their actions on it."

And, as often happens with people of vision and commitment, Bill McLinn had proven his naysayers wrong, traveling throughout the world and adding value and inspiration with every performance.

But playing Mark Twain was a minor challenge compared to the one he was facing onstage that night. In the 1980s, to reveal to an audience that he was infected with the HIV virus could mean the end of his career. Or the end of his relationship with his beloved wife's family, who were Japanese. In Japan, at that time, if a member of a family had AIDS, the entire family was ostracized, and Bill and his wife might never be allowed to return to Japan.

And yet Bill knew that he must embrace his challenge and reach out to others. Maybe he could play a small part in increasing the world's understanding of the reality of the AIDS epidemic. This was Bill's vision. The prospect of providing such a service to humanity outweighed his fear of professional ostracism and family discomfort. He cut through his story and let the truth be known.

Within a month of each other, Treya Killam Wilber and Bill McLinn passed over to the other side.

Up to the last breath, and now beyond, they continually inspire all who knew them with their passion, their caring, their humor, and their commitment to truth. Treya and Bill were able to live fully because they had faced death with a warrior spirit. In the heartbreak of their deaths we may find solace in the gift they have left. As in the old Sufi saying, "When the heart weeps for what it has lost, the spirit laughs for what it has found."

There are many times in my life when my story wants to hold me back. Having a compelling vision sharpens my sword, allowing me to cut through that story and courageously step forward. Although I have visions for specific areas of my life, I have a simple general one that has helped me keep my sword sharp—I envision a young child of the future standing strong and sturdy on the top of a lush green hill, silhouetted by the rising sun that she is facing. With her arms extended up to the heavens, a big, bold smile on her face, she is shouting "Yes!" to the Universe. And there is a tear of gratitude flowing down one cheek, saying thanks to the people of this time who dedicate their lives to preparing and nurturing the soil for that green earth and for her courageous spirit.

Sometimes when I'm about to face another audience, or maybe just another day, my stories grab me strongly from behind—"I'm feeling tired today, I'm not capable of doing this, I really have nothing new to offer." I simply breathe deeply, get centered, see that little child, and step forward, inviting whatever tears and fears I have to join me. If not now, when?

Each moment
the true warrior cuts through his story
and steps forth from his vision.
In this there is true power.

BE A WARRIOR

The great religious figures Jesus and Buddha, and heroes of nonviolence such as Gandhi and Martin Luther King, never drew a sword or packed a gun. And yet entire empires and cultures were changed forever as a result of their lives. They were true warriors, armed only with centered purpose, manifested through compassion and loving service for all humanity.

You can create such warriorship through daily practice. It is by living your centered purpose in the world, moment by moment. Let every red light, every mistake, every illness, every upset, and every injustice be a reminder of your higher purpose. Choose to be centered, and from this serenely grounded state, take effective action.

Centered purpose has power and vitality because it comes from within. It is not bullied by society's dictates nor belittled by your own frail need for approval. When your purpose is centered, you will feel an alignment of mind, body, and spirit. To find that purpose you must tune in to your natural gifts, talents, passions, and dreams. It is finding out who you really are, and living a life that demonstrates it.

Einstein was impassioned in his unwavering search for the principles of gravity, time, and space. Picasso followed an uninhibited love of color and images. Susan B. Anthony pursued justice and freedom despite vast odds. They were naturally able to parlay their gifts and passions into value for themselves and others.

When you follow your centered purpose, you are unconsciously supporting the Universe's purpose as well. Bucky Fuller called this principle "precession," and used the analogy of the honey bee. The honey bee's conscious purpose is to collect nectar from the flowers for its beehive. Unbeknownst to the bee, it is also participating in the Universe's grander plan—to cover the earth with flowers.

When you courageously live your centered purpose, you develop an immense feeling of gratitude for the deep inner peace that it provides. The natural outgrowth of this gratitude is discovering ways that your purpose adds value to others.

9

Walt Disney had a gift of imagination and fantasy. He went bankrupt five times in his pursuit of making a mouse into a mega-star. Now, for decades, Mickey Mouse and his supporting cast have brought joy to an entire world.

Former President Jimmy Carter loves cabinet-making and peace-making. In his retirement, he can be found banging nails in support of low-income housing one moment, and bringing warring nations to the negotiating table the next. So it is with the old man on a park bench sharing witty tales of wisdom with a wide-eyed kid. Or, the skilled entrepreneur organizing the community to support the end of hunger. Or the doctor and nurse giving their free time to perform eye surgery on the blind in Bangladesh. Or simply the young child dancing her dance and singing her song, uplifting whoever happens to be around.

Even though one gift may be lost, there is always another in its stead. Christopher Reeve, a talented actor who brought Superman back to the silver screen, became even more heroic in real life when he became a quadriplegic in an equestrian jumping accident. His tireless commitment to spinal cord research and to his own per-sonal healing, and his return to acting, writing, and directing, is an immense gift of inspiration to all who struggle daily with their own stories of limitation. It is phenomenal that he would be able to give so much after so much was taken away. Christopher Reeve is a man with the warrior spirit.

May we each find the courage to cut through our own stories, find the special gift that we are, and present it to the world. May our warrior spirits awaken!

I know I am Centered when:

- *I am balanced and stable.*
- *I am breathing deeply from my belly.*
- *I am relaxed, calm, and focused.*
- *I am aware, internally and externally.*
- *I am appreciative of myself and others.*
- *I am feeling my emotions—and learning from them.*
- *I am compassionate and connected to others and to my environment.*
- *I am able to receive and give sincere acknowledgement.*
- *I am energized by purpose.*
- *I am bigger than my story.*
- *I am unattached to the outcome of a situation.*
- *I am having fun and laughing often.*

Afterword

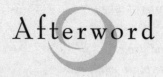

Thank you for allowing me to share some of my journey to center with you. You are on your own journey, traveling freely, by choice. If some of my stories have been meaningful, maybe it is because they are a mirror to your own stories, a juncture where our paths have converged.

Walt Whitman captures the joyful essence of the journey to center in "Song of the Open Road":

> *Afoot and light-hearted I take to the open road,*
> *Healthy, free, the world before me,*
> *The long brown path before me leading wherever I choose.*

> *Henceforth I ask not good-fortune, I myself am good-fortune,*
> *Henceforth I whimper no more, postpone no more, need nothing,*
> *Strong and content, I travel the open road.*

> *I inhale great draughts of space,*
> *The east and the west are mine, and the north and the south are mine.*

> *I am larger, better than I thought,*
> *I did not know I held so much goodness.*

ABOUT THE AUTHOR

Thomas Crum is an internationally known author, seminar leader, and martial artist. He is co-founder and president of Aiki Works, Inc. He leads seminars and training for organizations such as Walt Disney, Lucent Technologies, Georgia Pacific, Interface, and McDonald's. His work has taken him to many places throughout the world, including Russia, Northern Ireland, and South Africa.

A former educator and systems analyst, Tom co-founded, along with John Denver, the Windstar Foundation, an educational center on appropriate technology for a sustainable future. Tom also co-founded the Aspen Academy of Martial and Healing Arts.

He is the author of the book, *The Magic of Conflict,* and many audio and video programs dealing with conflict, stress management, and peak performance.

Tom is co-recipient of the American Society of Training and Development (ASTD) Vision Award for Performance Improvement for his role in the design and facilitation of Ashland Chemical's Simply the Best program, a multi-year program for management.

Tom also works as a peak performance coach for both professional and amateur athletes. His residential programs include week-long ski seminars in Aspen, Colorado, in the winter and golfing seminars in the summer.

For more information on Thomas Crum's products and programs, contact:

AIKI WORKS, INC.

P.O. Box 7845	or	P.O. Box 251
Aspen, CO 81612		Victor, NY 14564
(970)925-7099		(716)924-7302
Fax: (970)925-4532		Fax: (716)924-2799

Ancient pond
A frog jumps
And great silence

—BASHO